The Self-Care Cookbook

A **HOLISTIC APPROACH** TO
COOKING, EATING, AND LIVING WELL

DR. FRANK ARDITO

SURREY
BOOKS

AN AGATE IMPRINT

CHICAGO

Printed in China

Photos on pages iv, 6, 30, 58, 86, 124, 152, 174, 200, 226, 250 by iStock.com/Ondine32
All other photography by Zhao Photography
Recipe development and culinary consultation by Stacey Ballis
Art direction by Alice Zhao and Jared Zhao
Food styling by Alice Zhao, Jared Zhao, Stacey Ballis, and Bill Thurmond

The graphic on page 2 is adapted from the Prevention Through Wellness model © Dr. Francis Ardito for The Wellness Registry. All rights reserved. Find more information at www.mywellnessregistry.com.

The Self-Care Cookbook
ISBN 13: 978-1-57284-229-8
ISBN 10: 1-57284-229-6
eISBN 13: 978-1-57284-802-3
eISBN 10: 1-57284-802-2
First printing: November 2017

Surrey Books is an imprint of Agate Publishing. Agate books are available in bulk at discount prices. For more information, visit agatepublishing.com.

I would like to dedicate this book to my dear friend, life coach, and author-extraordinaire, Stacey Ballis. In addition to being the architect of each scrumptious recipe, chief culinary consultant, and senior food stylist, she is someone who truly espouses what it means to live and be well. Anyone who knows Stacey knows that, notwithstanding the very short list of aforementioned talents, she is someone who is simply brilliant and charming, authentically passionate, uncompromisingly available, and relentlessly supportive. Without Stacey and the countless hours of dedicated energy that she poured into each and every page, this book would simply not exist.

I would also like to acknowledge all those who have empowered me to live well and to all those who struggle with self-care—this one's for you!

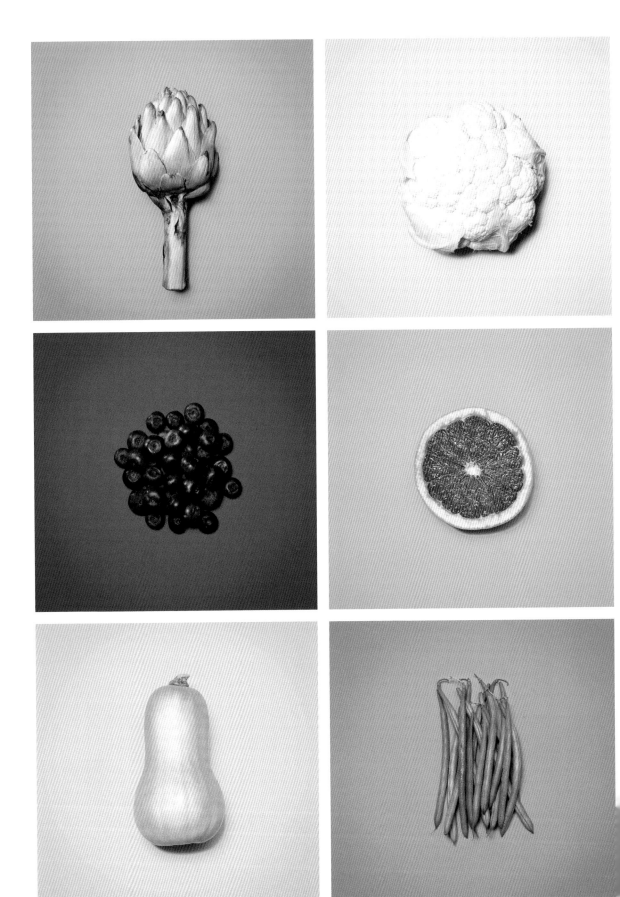

Contents

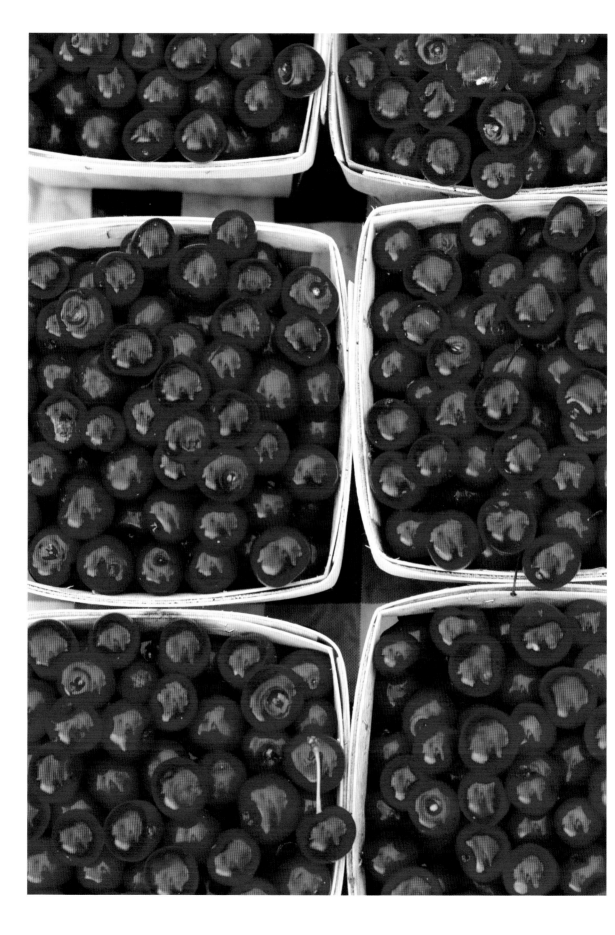

Introduction

I call this book *The Self-Care Cookbook* because most cookbooks are, at their core, essentially about cooking for other people—about feeding your family, getting dinner on the table for your spouse or partner, hosting holidays or celebrations, or exploring a different culture. While all of that is a part of this book, I wanted to underscore that this cookbook is about *you*.

It is, first and foremost, a cookbook. If your current feelings about your personal wellness are that you just don't have the bandwidth to even think about it, but you love great food and want to add new dishes to your repertoire, this book is still for you. You can skip the rest of this introduction, go straight to the recipes, and enjoy the variety of delicious options that await you.

But if you want to support your interest in wellness through food and cooking, then I hope you'll be as excited as I am by this new culinary approach to self-care.

WHAT IS WELLNESS?

These days, concepts regarding well-being are everywhere. We are inundated with the words—*wellness, health, dieting, weight loss, exercise*—but the definitions of each are vast. Of all of these, *wellness* wins the prize for the most misunderstood. A "wellness visit" can mean a doctor's appointment, a spa treatment, or checking in on someone elderly during a weather crisis. Dog food? There's a brand called Wellness. Even funeral homes use the word *wellness* to describe after-life care. All of this begs an important question: What is wellness, *really*?

At its core, wellness does indeed have an important meaning. The easiest way to wrap your head around it is to consider the difference between wellness and health. Health is an outcome—sometimes the result of choices, good or bad; sometimes the result of benefit or misfortune; sometimes the result of positive or negative genetics. Blood pressure, weight, and cholesterol levels are all examples of markers to help define one's health. Health is *not* always a choice. Wellness, on the other hand, is *always* a choice. It is the things you *choose* to do to enrich your life—enrolling in a class to learn

> Health is *not* always a choice. Wellness, on the other hand, is *always* a choice.

something new, going for a walk or a workout, or attending a faith-based service or a holiday celebration with friends and family. These are all ways to enhance your well-being, and they are all ways to improve aspects of your existence. True wellness is multidimensional and enormously empowering—not just from a physical perspective, which is often the first inference we make when we hear about wellness, but in a more complex and all-encompassing way.

The Wellness Registry, an organization I founded that awards the world's first consumer wellness certification, created a model (see below) for empowering wellness. Called *Prevention through Wellness*, it was created to put you in control of your complete personal wellness. You get to call the shots—you choose what is most important to you. It is much more than the simple "mind, body, and spirit" premise we have all seen. It defines 10 dimensions of you—and it gives you 10 choices for things you can choose to do to be well. Please note that the words on the left side indicate your health dimensions, and those along the right represent your wellness choices.

PREVENTION THROUGH WELLNESS

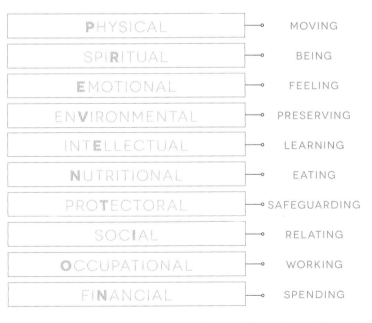

PHYSICAL	MOVING
SPIRITUAL	BEING
EMOTIONAL	FEELING
ENVIRONMENTAL	PRESERVING
INTELLECTUAL	LEARNING
NUTRITIONAL	EATING
PROTECTORAL	SAFEGUARDING
SOCIAL	RELATING
OCCUPATIONAL	WORKING
FINANCIAL	SPENDING

P · R · E · V · E · N · T · I · O · N

Adapted from the Prevention through Wellness model © Dr. Francis Ardito for The Wellness Registry. All rights reserved. www.mywellnessregistry.com

WHY I WROTE THIS BOOK

There have been hundreds of books written about health and wellness and thousands of published cookbooks. I had no interest in duplicating either of these. So, I asked myself a basic question: *What if?* What if there was a book that connected the dots between self-care and food; one that provided you not only with delicious recipes but also showed you which ones complement each aspect of your well-being? What if there was a resource to help you choose the foods that best support whatever it is that *you* are currently focused on for *your* personal wellness? And most importantly, what if the recipes in that book were easy for anyone to master and so delicious that the person cooking them would never hesitate to incorporate them into his or her life?

This book is not about dieting; it is about your diet. This book is not about dieting; it is about your diet. These are not the same thing. "Dieting" is about what you are limited to—a narrowly focused program of eating for a specific outcome, and these days, that almost always refers to a weight-loss program. While the majority of the recipes in this book will seamlessly fit into a dieting or weight-loss regimen, that isn't my focus. This book is about wellness and your relationship with food. It is about understanding how to eat "well" based upon *your* goals, *your* plans, *your* aspirations.

I believe that holistic wellness is about complete balance. Sometimes you need to cook and eat in a way that allows you to impact aspects of your physical self. Sometimes you need to cook and eat in a way that strengthens your social relationships, or even in a way that addresses how and what you eat during your workday. It is about recognizing that your relationship with food is constantly evolving, and I want to empower you to make choices in real time. On the road to wellness, there is no "right" path.

As someone who has devoted his career to training others in how to help people achieve personal wellness, I came to a shocking realization. One of the most important parts of our daily lives is our relationship with food. Studies have suggested that we make over 200 decisions about food every day! I'm not a particularly natural cook, and so, while my eating was always fine for my nutritional needs, I wasn't sure that my relationship with food was doing all it could for me in my own personal wellness journey.

It made me wonder: Could there be a cookbook where the cooking and eating was specifically aligned with the 10 aspects of personal wellness? Could I create a tool that was, at its core, designed for people just like me, who are committed to their wellness and want their eating and cooking to reflect that commitment? Could someone who isn't a cook write a cookbook? I knew the wellness part, and I knew the nutrition part, but I didn't have the recipes or skills to know how to put that into a cookbook.

Luckily for me, I did have a friend who had those skills! Stacey Ballis is a novelist, cookbook author, and food writer who has been developing recipes for decades. I have known Stacey for over 20 years and have eaten much of her delicious food. I reached out to her to see if she would be willing to be my culinary consultant and recipe developer for this project, and she agreed. In the process of working with Stacey on the recipes and techniques for this book, my own cooking and eating began to naturally align with my own wellness journey. It has become a true road map to the way I cook and eat, and I believe that I am more "well" today as a result. And I believe that it will work the same for you.

HOW TO USE THIS BOOK

As you may have already noticed, this book isn't set up like other cookbooks. Instead of grouping recipes by what kind of dish they are or what time of day you eat them, each chapter in this book is dedicated to one of the 10 dimensions of your well-being.

Each chapter contains 13 recipes that support a particular dimension of your wellness, which corresponds with the diagram on page 2. Each chapter offers a wide array of dishes so you can find something to suit your needs and lifestyle, including appetizers, soups, salads, mains, and desserts. The sides and mains for each category of wellness offer a variety of options to suit your preferences, including pastas, grains, all manner of meat proteins, and vegetarian options. In the introduction to each chapter, I define the relevant dimension of wellness and explain how it interacts with both cooking *and* eating the recipes in that chapter.

Need to be mentally sharp for an upcoming round of exams, job interviews, or a big project? Check out the recipes in the chapter

A balanced life includes celebratory foods in harmony with foods that are supportive of health.

on intellectual wellness, full of ingredients that are known to positively impact brain health, matched with cooking techniques that support neuroplasticity. Are you stressed or upset? Peruse the delicious and indulgent comfort food choices in the emotional wellness chapter. Looking for ways to eat on a budget? The financial wellness chapter gives you tasty food creations that are pennywise.

Let's face it: you can choose not to diet, you can choose not to exercise, but you must eat. So, why not choose to eat *well*? Unlike diet cookbooks, I recognize that sometimes eating well means eating foods that some people would call "bad." I don't believe in bad food. I believe in delicious food. I don't believe in restrictions or denial. I believe in moderation. I believe that your complete wellness as it relates to cooking and eating includes both ends of the spectrum, from creative ideas for fresh, light dishes that fuel our bodies for activity and strength to wonderful indulgences that embrace fat and sugar and acknowledge their positive impact on our souls. A balanced life includes celebratory foods in harmony with foods that are supportive of health, and I believe that a part of your wellness is deciding, at any given moment, which you want or need most. *The Self-Care Cookbook* is a new way of looking at the intersection of cooking, eating, and wellness, and I hope that you will enjoy using it as much as I have enjoyed creating it for you.

DR. FRANK ARDITO

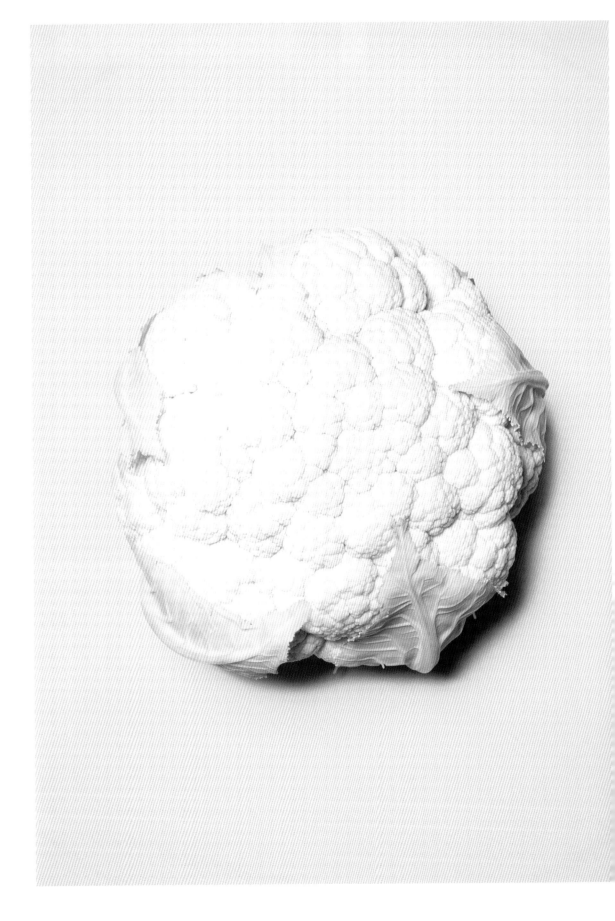

CHAPTER 1: Physical Wellness

PHYSICAL WELLNESS IS ABOUT **MOVING**. Your heart and lungs work in concert to provide nutrient delivery to every part of you, and your muscles utilize that fuel to allow you to move. Similarly, every other system of your body has structures and functions that support movement. Physical activities such as walking, housework, and taking the stairs instead of the elevator are excellent ways to enhance your health but will not necessarily make you physically fit. In contrast, exercises such as jogging, weight training, and group classes will make you more physically fit, but they will not necessarily make you healthy. For example, a distance runner may be very fit but may also suffer from repetitive trauma injuries. Wellness is about choices, and whatever you choose, be sure to move!

Wellness is about choices, and whatever you choose, be sure to move!

COOKING for physical well-being means *moving* as much as possible while you prepare your meals—safety permitting! This might include manually cutting your fruits and vegetables, standing up during food prep, and moving about the kitchen whenever possible. The more you move, the more you will enhance your physical well-being. One practical tip when you are cooking is to try to balance the amount of physical exertion between your right and left arms and legs. For example, if you typically use your right hand/arm to stir a sauce, then consider switching to your left. If you typically shift your body weight to your right leg while standing at the counter, shift it over to the left. Balance is the key!

EATING for physical well-being means eating foods that support how you choose to move. If you don't currently exercise but are physically active (or perhaps not), then enjoy the foods in this chapter in moderation. Consider eating a half portion and saving the rest for later or sharing it with a workout partner. If you are an avid exerciser or athlete, then fuel up and enjoy full portions of the tasty selections in this chapter. Each of them is loaded with energy-producing macronutrients: complex carbohydrates and fats and high-quality proteins for tissue growth and repair after strenuous physical exertion. For most people, the key to eating for physical well-being is to identify the amount of food that you will be able to ultimately burn off through your physical activity of choice.

French Carrot Salad

The few ingredients in this salad make for a very special dish, and the colors are gorgeous on any plate. Carrots, usually known for their ability to improve and protect eye health, are also full of vitamin A and potassium, not to mention fiber and beta-carotene, which are two of your best weapons against colon cancer. Parsley contains powerful antioxidants and is a great source of vitamin C.

5 tablespoons fruity extra virgin olive oil
2 tablespoons red wine vinegar
½ teaspoon kosher salt, plus more to taste
1 teaspoon dried oregano or thyme
½ teaspoon Dijon mustard

1½ pounds carrots, peeled and grated
  (see Note)
¼ cup chopped fresh flat-leaf parsley
Freshly ground black pepper, to taste

To make the dressing, put the olive oil, vinegar, salt, oregano, and mustard into a small jar and shake well. (It's great to make this recipe when you notice your mustard jar is down to its last dregs; you can mix the dressing right in the jar.) It does not have to be completely emulsified, just well mixed.

In a large bowl, toss together the carrots and parsley until the parsley is well distributed. Add three-quarters of the dressing and give the salad a good mix. Taste and add salt and pepper as needed, and more dressing, if desired. Store any leftover dressing in the fridge for up to 1 week. Serve the salad chilled or at room temperature.

NOTE: Please do not use pre-shredded carrots in this recipe. While they are a great time-saver for many things, like soups or stews, the key to this salad is the sweet juiciness that is achieved with freshly grated carrots—it is really worth the effort. Use the grater blade on your food processor, the large side of your box grater, or even that fancy spiralizer if you have one!

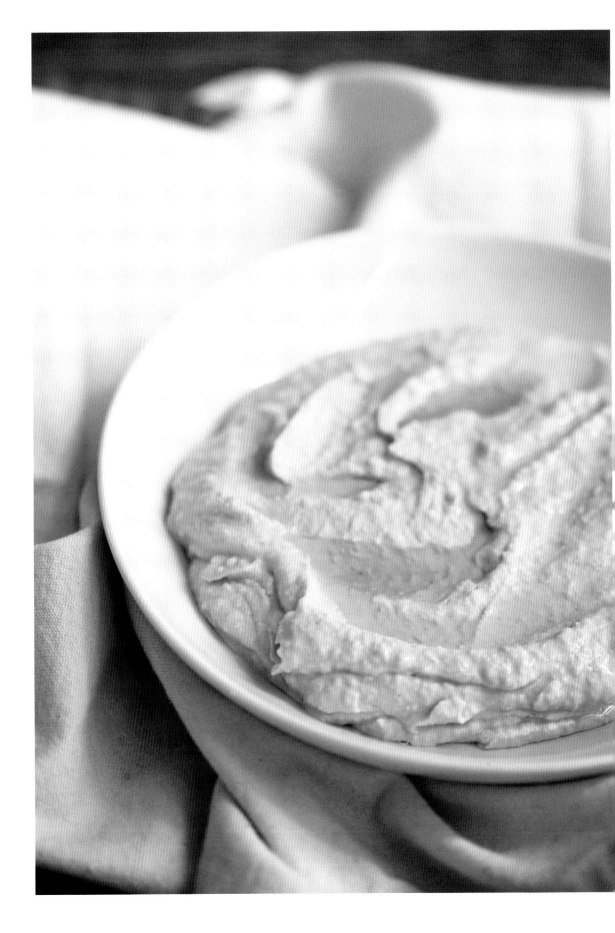

Classic Hummus

SERVES 8

From a physical perspective, this hummus packs a wallop. The beans and tahini are both protein bombs, and keeping this versatile dip around is a great way to grab a snack that will fill you up and fuel you for the rest of the day. I encourage you to make this at home instead of buying it at a store, as store-bought brands tend to be high in sodium and preservatives. There are many recipes out there, and most will tell you to use dried chickpeas. Their preparation, while worth it, can be time consuming. This version uses canned chickpeas, saving you time, and is just as delicious. Buy high-quality organic and low-sodium canned chickpeas if you can find them.

1 teaspoon kosher salt, plus more to taste
3 tablespoons freshly squeezed lemon juice
2 (15-ounce) cans chickpeas, drained and
   rinsed
1¼ cups tahini

½ cup cold water, plus more as needed
Freshly ground black pepper, to taste
Hot sauce, to taste (optional)
Good-quality extra virgin olive oil, for serving

In a small bowl or cup, dissolve the salt into the lemon juice. This helps distribute the salt flavor throughout the dish and prevents anyone from biting into a salt bomb!

In a high-powered blender, combine the chickpeas and the salted lemon juice. Pulse a few times to break up the chickpeas and begin to make a paste. Add the tahini and purée until the mixture just begins to form a smoother, cohesive paste. With the machine running, slowly add the water and continue blending until the mixture is very smooth and creamy, almost fluffy, 2 to 4 minutes. You might not need all of the water, depending on how liquid the tahini was. If the hummus becomes too thick, drizzle in more water.

Taste and add salt and pepper as needed, and hot sauce, if using. Pulse to blend.

Transfer to a serving bowl, drizzle with olive oil, and serve.

NOTE: This recipe is as basic as it gets. Dress it up to suit your preferences. For example, you can add ½ to 4 cloves of garlic. I also recommend experimenting with spices such as cumin and smoked paprika; herb blends like za'atar; and fresh herbs like parsley, mint, and dill. While this recipe works best in a high-powered blender, you can use your food processor as well. If you prefer chunkier hummus, pulse instead of purée and use less water.

Store any leftovers in a covered container in the fridge for up to 3 days. The hummus will taste best if it comes to room temperature before serving.

Chilled Cucumber Soup

SERVES 6

This soup, an easy, elegant start to a meal, is a healthy bowl of bright flavors: the Greek yogurt is terrific source of protein, calcium, and probiotics (which help keep your gut healthy); the almonds have protein, fiber, and vitamin E; and the cucumbers, a little-known superfood that helps keep you hydrated, are a wonderful source of potassium and electrolytes and have been shown to raise antioxidant levels.

3 large English (or hothouse/seedless) cucumbers, peeled
1 teaspoon white wine vinegar or sherry
1 tablespoon freshly squeezed lemon juice
1 teaspoon kosher salt, plus more to taste
1 cup full-fat plain Greek yogurt
½ teaspoon lemon zest
3 green onions, chopped (white and pale-green parts only)
1 small shallot, minced
4 tablespoons chopped fresh dill, divided

¼ cup + 3 tablespoons sliced Marcona almonds, divided
¼ teaspoon freshly ground white pepper, plus more to taste
1 cup homemade or store-bought low-sodium vegetable stock or broth, or less as needed
2 tablespoons extra virgin olive oil, plus more for garnish
1 tablespoon chopped fresh flat-leaf parsley, for garnish

Halve the cucumbers lengthwise and scrape out the seeds with a spoon. Dice one of the halves into ¼-inch cubes and set aside in the fridge. Chop the remaining cucumbers into large chunks and transfer to a blender.

In a small bowl, mix together the vinegar and lemon juice, dissolve the salt into this mixture, and then add it to the blender. Add the yogurt, lemon zest, green onions, shallot, 3 tablespoons of the dill, ¼ cup of the almonds, and the white pepper. Pulse a few times to break down the cucumbers. When the mixture is chunky, purée it on medium-high speed until very smooth. Reduce the speed to medium and, with the machine running, slowly drizzle in the vegetable stock until the soup is as smooth as possible and has the consistency of heavy cream. You may not need all of the stock.

Cover the blender and set aside at room temperature to allow the flavors to meld, 30 minutes to 1 hour. If it is a particularly warm day, chill the blended mixture in the fridge for the first 20 minutes of this resting period. While the soup rests, coarsely chop the remaining 3 tablespoons of almonds and set aside.

After the soup has rested (and is room temperature, if you put it in the fridge at first), pulse it a couple times to remix. Taste and add salt and white pepper as needed. Chill the finished soup in a bowl or pitcher for at least 2 hours.

Just before serving, add the diced cucumber and the olive oil and stir well to combine. Transfer the soup to serving bowls, and garnish each bowl with the chopped almonds, the remaining tablespoon of dill, and the parsley. Add a few drops of oil to each bowl. Serve immediately.

NOTE: If your soup is seasoned well but still lacks punch, add either more lemon juice or more vinegar, ½ teaspoon at a time, until you are happy with the balance. You can make this up to 2 days in advance; just be sure to stir well to reblend the mixture before serving.

Salmon Steaks with Asian Marinade

SERVES 4

Some say that the farmed salmon found at grocery stores does not have the same health benefits as wild-caught salmon. This isn't the reason we specify wild-caught here—we just think it's more delicious! Oily fishes like salmon are low-calorie sources of protein and have high levels of omega-3s. If you aren't a salmon fan, this works equally well with tuna steaks or halibut. Coconut aminos are an interesting substitute for soy sauce, great if you know someone who is gluten-free or soy-free, but they also add an interesting base note here. If you can't find coconut aminos, you can substitute low-sodium soy sauce or tamari.

⅓ cup homemade or store-bought low-sodium vegetable stock
1 teaspoon lime zest (see Note)
1 tablespoon freshly squeezed lime juice
1 tablespoon amber agave nectar
2 tablespoons coconut aminos
1 tablespoon hoisin sauce
1 teaspoon minced garlic

1 teaspoon grated fresh ginger
Pinch red pepper flakes
Pinch five-spice powder
3 tablespoons grapeseed oil, divided
4 (8-ounce) wild-caught salmon steaks, skinned
Kosher salt and freshly ground black pepper, to taste

To make the marinade, mix together the stock, lime zest, lime juice, agave nectar, coconut aminos, hoisin sauce, garlic, ginger, red pepper flakes, five-spice powder, and 2 tablespoons of the oil. Transfer the marinade to a gallon-size zip-top bag. Add the salmon steaks and let them marinate in the fridge for 30 minutes. Do not let the fish sit for longer than 30 minutes, as the acids in the marinade will begin to cook the delicate fish and your finished dish will have a mushy texture.

Preheat the oven to 400°F. Remove the salmon from the marinade, reserving the liquid, and pat the salmon very dry with paper towels. Season with salt and pepper. In an ovenproof, nonstick skillet, heat the remaining tablespoon of oil over high heat until it shimmers.

Add the salmon to the pan. Cook on one side for 1 minute without moving, which should make a nice golden crust. Flip the salmon and cook for 1 more minute to get the crust on the other side.

Add the reserved marinade to the pan and bring it to a boil. Transfer the pan to the oven and bake for 6 minutes (for medium rare) to 10 minutes (if you prefer it cooked through). Serve immediately.

> **NOTE:** When working with limes, always zest before you juice; it is much easier to get the zest off of a whole fruit. Since limes can be a bit hard to juice, try rolling the whole fruit on the counter with firm pressure from your palm back and forth a couple of times. This breaks up some of the fruit cells inside the lime and makes it easier to juice.

Roast Pork Loin with Pomegranate Salsa

SERVES 4

Pork loin is a wonderful lean meat and is beautifully brightened with this take on salsa. And while I recommend it with pork, the salsa is a great partner for just about any meat or fish you choose. The pomegranate and cucumber bring many antioxidants to the party, while the parsley and lime add some vitamin C as well.

⅓ cup minced red onion
Freshly squeezed juice of 1 lime
1 teaspoon red wine vinegar
½ teaspoon kosher salt, plus more to taste
1 tablespoon pomegranate molasses
2 cups pomegranate seeds (see Note)
1 cup finely diced seedless cucumber

2 serrano chiles, seeds removed and finely minced
¼ cup finely chopped fresh flat-leaf parsley
Freshly ground black pepper, to taste
1 tablespoon grapeseed or canola oil
2 pounds pork loin

To make the salsa, soak the onion in a small bowl of cold, salted water for 10 minutes. This will help take some of the harsh bite out of the onion. Drain the onion completely and return to the bowl. In a separate small bowl, combine the lime juice, vinegar, and salt. Stir to combine, then add the pomegranate molasses and give it another good stir. Add this mixture to the bowl of minced onion, mix well, and let sit for 10 minutes.

Stir in the pomegranate seeds, cucumber, chiles, and parsley. Taste and add salt and pepper as needed, then set aside.

In a large sauté pan set over medium-high heat, heat the oil until it shimmers. Season the pork well on all sides with salt and pepper. Add the pork, fat-side down, and sear until it is golden brown, 2 to 3 minutes per side. Cover the pan, reduce the heat to low, and cook for 25 to 30 minutes, until an instant-read thermometer inserted into the thickest part of the meat registers 150°F.

Transfer the pork to a wire rack and let it rest, uncovered, for 10 to 15 minutes. Carve into ½-inch-thick slices and serve with the pomegranate salsa.

> **NOTE**: Many stores now carry pomegranate seeds already prepped, but if yours does not, buy 2 whole pomegranates. Halve them and use a wooden spoon to thwack them over a large bowl to get the seeds out. Pick out any of the white pith that has fallen into your bowl before proceeding. Pomegranate molasses can usually be found in the same aisle as honey and sugar-based molasses. If your regular grocery store doesn't carry it, check Middle Eastern grocery stores.

Poached Chicken with Broccoli Pesto

SERVES 4

While we all appreciate that the white meat of chicken is high in protein and low in fat and calories, it's also low in flavor and easy to make badly. But, it is possible to make chicken breasts that are both delicious and healthy. Poaching is an easy, effective way to keep chicken breasts moist, and it creates a tender base for this vibrant and surprising riff on pesto. Broccoli is one of the most nutrient-dense vegetables you can eat.

2 quarts cold water
2 cups homemade or low-sodium store-bought chicken stock
4 (8-ounce) boneless, skinless chicken breasts
2 tablespoons grapeseed oil
½ small yellow onion, chopped
2 small cloves garlic, minced
½ pound fresh or frozen broccoli florets, cooked

¼ cup toasted pine nuts or almond slivers (see Note on page 159)
½ cup loosely packed fresh basil leaves
½ cup grated Parmesan, plus more for garnish
Pinch red pepper flakes (optional)
4 tablespoons extra virgin olive oil, plus more for garnish
Kosher salt and freshly ground black pepper, to taste

In a small stockpot, mix the cold water and stock. Add the chicken breasts. You want to start the chicken cold so that it heats at the same pace as the water. Bring to a boil over high heat. Boil for 6 minutes, then cover the pot, turn off the heat, and leave the pot on the burner. Let the chicken continue to cook in the covered pot for 45 minutes. No peeking! You want to retain the heat, and lifting the lid lets steam and heat escape.

While the chicken is poaching, make the pesto. In a large skillet set over medium-high heat, heat the grapeseed oil until it shimmers. Add the onion and cook until it is translucent. Add the garlic and cook for 1 minute, watching carefully so that it doesn't color; burnt garlic is very bitter. Add the broccoli and cook, stirring frequently, until the broccoli is very soft and can be easily broken apart with a spoon. You are going for mushy here, so that the broccoli will blend well and be soft.

Transfer the broccoli mixture to the bowl of a food processor. Add the pine nuts and pulse until the mixture is a coarse mash. Add the basil, Parmesan, and red pepper flakes, if using, and pulse to mix. With the machine running, slowly add the olive oil. Turn off the processor, taste and add salt and pepper as needed, and set aside.

To serve, slice the poached chicken breasts into ½-inch-thick slices and generously spoon the broccoli pesto over them. Garnish with a drizzle of olive oil and a sprinkle of Parmesan, and serve immediately.

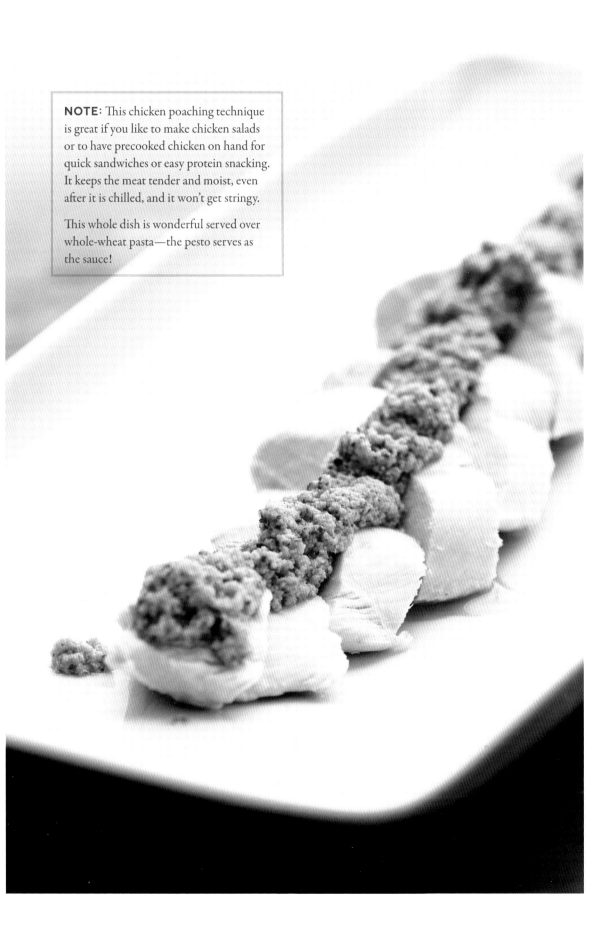

NOTE: This chicken poaching technique is great if you like to make chicken salads or to have precooked chicken on hand for quick sandwiches or easy protein snacking. It keeps the meat tender and moist, even after it is chilled, and it won't get stringy.

This whole dish is wonderful served over whole-wheat pasta—the pesto serves as the sauce!

Marinated Flank Steak with Kale Salsa Verde

Flank steak is a terrific lean cut for when you are craving beef but don't want to indulge in a high-fat meal. Kale is the most popular superfood at the moment, which means we are all starting to get a little sick of it in salads. This hearty garnish is a great new way to think about kale, using it almost as a leafy herb and seasoning.

½ cup soy sauce
3 tablespoons vegetable oil
1 small yellow onion, chopped
3 cloves garlic, minced
2 tablespoons minced fresh ginger

2 tablespoons firmly packed dark brown sugar
Pinch red pepper flakes
½ cup pineapple juice
1 (1½–2-pound) flank steak
Kale Salsa Verde, for serving (recipe follows)

To make the marinade, mix together the soy sauce, oil, onion, garlic, ginger, brown sugar, red pepper flakes, and pineapple juice in a small bowl. Transfer to a gallon-size zip-top bag. Add the steak and let it marinate in the fridge for 8 to 24 hours.

Preheat a charcoal grill. If using a gas grill, preheat to medium high.

Place the steak on the grill, directly over the flame, and cook for about 4 minutes on each side, or until an instant-read thermometer inserted into the thickest part of the meat reads 130°F, for medium rare. Remove the steak from the grill and let it rest for 10 minutes.

Slice the steak thinly across the grain on a sharp diagonal, divide the pieces into 4 equal portions, and serve each portion with the Kale Salsa Verde on top or on the side.

> **NOTE**: While it is preferable to cook this steak on the grill, you can still do this in your oven. Just preheat the broiler to high and place the steak, on a broiler pan, on the oven's top rack. Cook for 4 to 5 minutes on each side for medium rare, then let the steak rest per the recipe's instructions.

Kale Salsa Verde

3 cups tightly packed torn kale leaves, washed
    well and ribs removed
½ cup fresh flat-leaf parsley leaves
¼ cup fresh mint leaves
1 tablespoon fresh marjoram leaves
1 tablespoon capers
½ tablespoon lemon zest
2 tablespoons freshly squeezed lemon juice
1 small clove garlic
½ teaspoon smoked paprika
½ cup extra virgin olive oil
Kosher salt and freshly ground black pepper,
    to taste

Bring a large pot of salted water to a boil
over medium-high heat. Add the kale and
cook until tender, about 3 minutes. Drain
well and rinse under cold running water until the kale is no longer warm to the touch.

Transfer the kale to the bowl of a food
processor. Add the parsley, mint, marjoram, capers, lemon zest and juice, garlic,
paprika, and oil. Pulse until the mixture
is a coarse, chunky paste. Taste and add
salt and pepper as needed. Transfer to a
serving bowl.

> **NOTE:** If you aren't a kale fan, try this
> recipe with mustard, turnip, or beet greens.
> For a milder version, use Swiss chard or
> spinach. If you can't find fresh marjoram,
> substitute fresh oregano.

High-Protein Shake

I don't advocate using shakes or smoothies as meal replacements more than once or twice a week. Your best bet for good satiation is to actually eat meals; the act of chewing and swallowing helps you eat at a nice, slow pace so that your body has time to recognize that it's full—you will be far more satisfied. However, sometimes you need a convenient format. This high-protein shake has a lot of calcium. The fact that it tastes a bit like an oatmeal, peanut butter, and banana cookie is a bonus! This is also a good pre- and post-workout snack. Drink one-third to one-half of the shake 15 to 20 minutes before your workout, and the rest right after. The healthy carbs will give you energy for the workout, and the protein will help you recover after.

2 tablespoons rolled oats
2 cups cold 2% milk, plus more as needed
1 medium ripe banana, cut into chunks
¼ cup vanilla Greek yogurt

¼ cup all-natural smooth peanut butter
1 heaping teaspoon agave syrup
1 teaspoon malted milk powder (optional)

Use a coffee grinder or food processor to very finely grind the oats. You are looking for something like a coarse powder. This is better than using premade oat flour, which is superfine and can get gummy.

In a medium bowl or measuring cup, stir the ground oats into the milk. Mix well, then set aside soak for 10 minutes to soften. Transfer the milk mixture to a blender. Add the banana, yogurt, peanut butter, agave syrup, and malted milk powder, if using. Blend on medium-high speed until very smooth. If the consistency is a bit too thick for your taste, add more milk, 1 tablespoon at a time, until you get the consistency you desire. Serve immediately.

> **NOTE:** If you are going to take this shake with you on the go, use frozen banana chunks to help keep the dairy cold. You can substitute the nut milk of your choice if you don't want to use cow's milk.
>
> Experiment with different nut butters to alter the flavor, change up your sweetener with honey or maple syrup, or even add instant espresso powder or cocoa powder for coffee or chocolate versions!

Chickpea and Pumpkin Stew

This hearty stew is a perfect blend of protein and healthy carbs, with plenty of fiber and, most important, plenty of flavor! Serve with crusty bread and a green salad for a complete meal that will keep vegetarians and meat eaters alike satisfied.

2 tablespoons peanut oil
1 large yellow onion, diced
2 ribs celery, diced
3 carrots, diced
2 cloves garlic, finely chopped
½ teaspoon grated fresh ginger
1 teaspoon ground cumin
1 teaspoon smoked paprika
3 cups homemade or store-bought low-sodium vegetable stock

½ cup farro
1 (1-pound) pumpkin or butternut squash, peeled and cut into 1-inch cubes
2 (15-ounce) cans chickpeas, drained and rinsed
Kosher salt and freshly ground black pepper, to taste
½ cup fresh flat-leaf parsley leaves
¼ cup chopped roasted peanuts, for garnish

In a Dutch oven set over medium-high heat, heat the oil until it shimmers. Reduce the heat to low. Add the onion, celery, and carrots and cook for 5 minutes, until the onion is translucent. Add the garlic, ginger, cumin, and paprika and cook, stirring constantly, for 1 minute. You want the mixture to be fragrant but not browned.

Add the stock, increase the heat to medium-high, and bring to a boil. Add the farro, stir, reduce the heat to medium, and cook, uncovered, for 15 minutes. Add the pumpkin and chickpeas. Simmer, uncovered, for 25 to 30 minutes, until the vegetables are soft and the farro is cooked al dente. Remove from the heat. Taste and add salt and pepper as needed.

When ready to serve, stir in the parsley. Portion the soup into bowls and serve hot garnished with the peanuts.

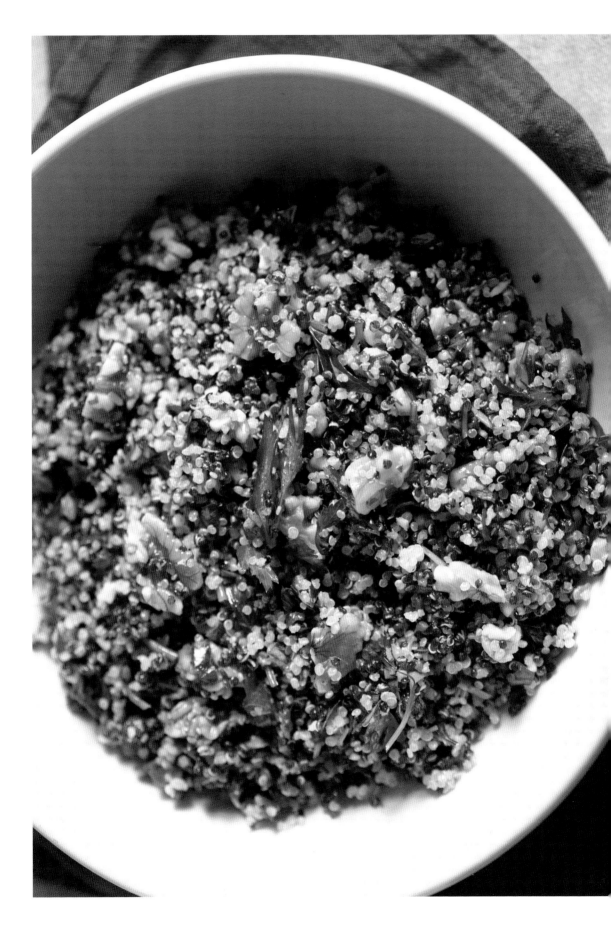

Quinoa Pilaf with Walnuts

Quinoa, a healthy grain substitute, has double the protein of most grains. When eaten regularly as part of a healthy diet, it has been shown to have positive effects on both blood sugar levels and blood pressure. Walnuts are one of the only plant-based sources of omega-3s, and they have higher levels of antioxidants than any other nut. This recipe doubles down on the walnuts, using both the whole nut and the oil. Walnut oil might seem like quite the luxury item, but it is terrific in salads or on top of cooked vegetables. Once you have a bottle in the house, you will find all sorts of uses for it.

1 cup raw quinoa (red, black, or a mixture)
2 cups water
½ teaspoon kosher salt, plus more to taste
3 tablespoons grapeseed oil
2 cups finely chopped yellow onion
1 tablespoon walnut oil

1 cup chopped roasted walnuts
1 teaspoon fresh thyme leaves
Freshly ground black pepper, to taste
2 tablespoons finely minced fresh flat-leaf
   parsley

Heat a large skillet over medium heat until it feels warm but not uncomfortable when you place your palm a couple inches above its surface. Add the quinoa and toast, gently swirling the skillet to keep the grains moving, until they are slightly deepened in color and smell a bit nutty. Remove the skillet from the heat and transfer the toasted quinoa to a bowl.

In a small saucepan set over high heat, bring the water and salt to a rolling boil. Add the toasted quinoa, reduce the heat to medium-high, and cook, uncovered, for a few minutes. Spoon out a few grains and taste to see if they are tender. The quinoa should pop between your teeth, be slightly al dente and not mushy, and not be crunchy or stick in your teeth. If it's not tender, continue cooking. While it is tempting to give you a time for this, every brand and type of quinoa responds differently, so it's best to read the package directions and start tasting the quinoa for proper doneness about 2 minutes before the package indicates. It might take as little as 12 or as many as 25 minutes. Remove from the heat and set aside.

In the same skillet you used to toast the quinoa, heat the grapeseed oil over medium-high heat until it shimmers. Add the onion and cook, stirring often, until it is very tender and slightly golden brown.

CONTINUED ▷

Quinoa Pilaf with Walnuts
CONTINUED

Reduce the heat to low, add the cooked quinoa, and stir with a fork. (As with rice or any grain, don't stir it with a spoon; it will clump and get gummy.) Add the walnut oil and toss lightly with a fork, then stir in the walnuts and thyme. Taste and add salt and pepper as needed.

Continue to gently heat until the pilaf is warmed through. Transfer it to a serving bowl, fold in the parsley, and serve.

NOTE: This toasting method will improve the flavor of all your quinoa dishes. If you cook with quinoa a lot, toast an entire package, remove the amount you need for this recipe, and store the rest in a sealed container in your pantry for up to six months.

If you want to make this a vegetarian entrée, add one can of chickpeas or white beans (drained and rinsed) to the onion mixture to bring some protein to the party. You may need to adjust the seasoning upwards by half.

Cauliflower Mash

Let me be very clear: this is not a recipe that tries to make cauliflower taste like potatoes. Potatoes taste like potatoes. Cauliflower tastes like cauliflower. However, there are times when you want a mild, buttery mash to go with your meat, but you either want to limit your carbs or save them for dessert. This is the mash for you. Cauliflower is actually richer in vitamins—especially vitamin C—than other brassicas (including broccoli!), making this a no-brainer. You'll be surprised at how such a small amount of butter can bring so much flavor to the dish.

1½–2 pounds cauliflower, cut into florets, core and leaves discarded
1½ teaspoons unsalted butter
Pinch ground nutmeg

½ teaspoon freshly ground black pepper, plus more to taste
Kosher salt, to taste

Bring a large pot of well-salted water to a boil over high heat. Add the cauliflower. Cook for at least 20 minutes, until completely soft. You should get no resistance at all when you press the florets with a spoon; the mash will have the wrong texture if you don't let it get soft enough.

Drain the cauliflower well and return to the pot; reduce the heat to low. Using a potato masher, thoroughly mash the cauliflower. Cook the mash, stirring constantly with a wooden spoon, for 3 to 4 minutes. You will notice liquid coming out of the mash. Continue to mash the cauliflower as the moisture cooks out. It is fine if the mixture begins to brown a little, but don't let it burn!

Remove the mash from the heat and stir in the butter, nutmeg, and pepper. Taste and add salt and pepper as needed. Serve hot.

Roasted Sweet Potatoes, Parsnips, and Pears

SERVES 8 AS A SIDE

Sweet potatoes are healthy and delicious. Their natural sweetness combined with their low glycemic index makes them a wonderful ingredient for diabetics and other people who are concerned about blood sugar. Parsnips, which people sometimes confuse for white carrots, are another secret superfood, with three B-complex vitamins, potassium, vitamin C, and plenty of fiber. The pears enhance the sweet flavor. I love this served with pork, but it also works with duck.

4 sweet potatoes, peeled
2 pounds parsnips, peeled
2 slightly underripe Bosc pears
3 tablespoons grapeseed oil

Kosher salt and freshly ground black pepper, to taste
3 sprigs fresh thyme
1 tablespoon white balsamic vinegar, for serving

Preheat the oven to 400°F.

Cut the sweet potatoes into large wedges, about 8 wedges per potato. Halve the parsnips lengthwise, and then halve each piece crosswise. Core the pears and cut them into thick wedges, leaving the skin on. All of the pieces of fruit and vegetables should be roughly the same size.

In a large bowl, toss the sweet potatoes, parsnips, and pears with the oil until everything is well coated. Add salt and pepper and toss again. Transfer the mixture to a 9 × 13-inch casserole dish, making sure the mixture is in a single layer. Add the thyme sprigs, tucking them into the mixture.

Bake, stirring occasionally, for 45 minutes, until the parsnips and potatoes are tender. Remove from the oven and discard the thyme sprigs. Drizzle with the balsamic vinegar and serve hot.

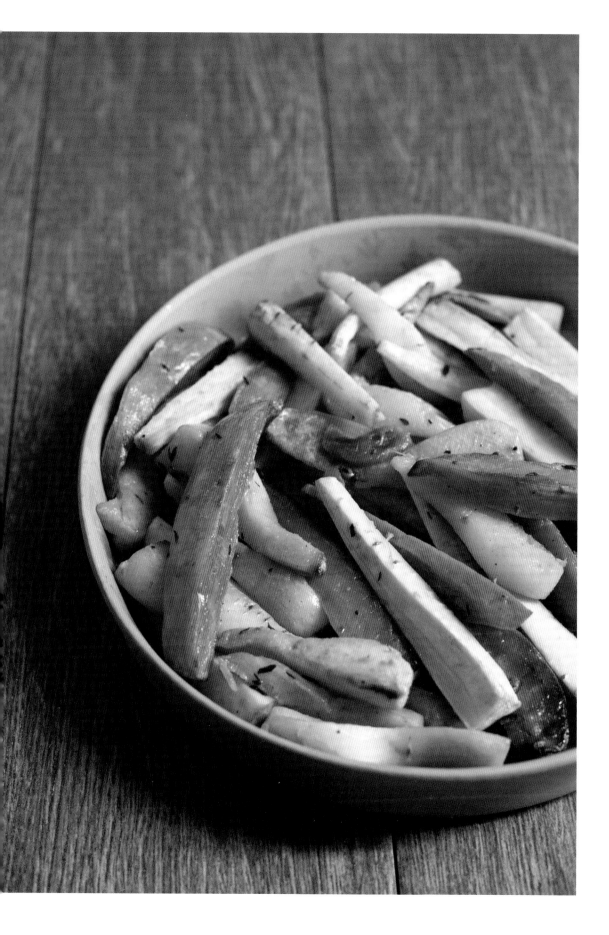

No-Bake Crustless Cheesecake with Balsamic Berries

SERVES 8

Traditional cheesecake is a calorie-bomb dessert, but the flavors are amazing and it does have a lot of protein. I wanted to get those wonderful flavors into a dessert with some healthful updates. First I eliminate the crust, so the filling can really shine. I've lightened it and brought some health to the party by replacing some of the traditional cream cheese and cream with Greek yogurt, which adds a wonderful tang to the dish. And by making it a no-bake option, it becomes a terrific dessert for summer. Bringing fresh berries and dried cherries into the mix also gives you an added burst of health benefits. As with any dessert in this book, the portions here are small but satisfying. Don't be tempted to adjust this recipe with low-fat versions of the cream cheese or yogurt, or to reduce the amount of cream. I believe that a small, rational portion of a full-fat dessert will satisfy you completely.

1¼ cups plain Greek yogurt
10 ounces cream cheese, fully softened
½ teaspoon vanilla paste

⅓ cup powdered sugar, sifted
1 cup heavy whipping cream
Balsamic Berries, for serving (recipe follows)

Set a mesh strainer over a large bowl, making sure there is plenty of space between the bottom of the strainer and the bottom of the bowl. Put the yogurt in the strainer, lightly cover it with plastic wrap, and transfer it to the fridge to chill for a minimum of 4 hours or as long as overnight. This strains off some of the liquid in the yogurt and gives it a consistency closer to the cream cheese. Since this no-bake cheesecake has no eggs to tighten up the mixture, this step is essential to ensure that you will be able to form the cheesecake.

Once the yogurt has chilled long enough, soak a large piece of cheesecloth in cold water for 3 minutes. Squeeze out the water so that the cheesecloth is just damp but not dripping wet. Fold the cloth in half and then in half again. Line a large mesh strainer with it and set it over a large bowl, then set it aside.

Remove the yogurt from the fridge and discard the liquid. Transfer the yogurt to a medium bowl. Add the cream cheese. With an electric handheld mixer, beat the yogurt and cream cheese on medium speed until well combined and fluffy. Add the vanilla paste and powdered sugar and beat until the mixture is smooth. You are using vanilla paste here because extract adds liquid to a mixture that is trying to be firm. (You can also use the scraped seeds from one vanilla pod.) Set this bowl aside.

In a separate bowl, whip the cream with your handheld mixer until soft peaks form, then carefully fold the whipped cream into the cream cheese–yogurt mixture until everything is well combined.

Spoon the mixture into the prepared strainer to catch the liquid that drains off. Again, make sure there is plenty of space between the strainer and the bottom of the bowl. Fold the cheesecloth loosely over the top of the mixture, lightly cover it with plastic wrap, and transfer to the fridge to chill for at least 8 hours or as long as overnight. The cheesecake is ready when you can press lightly on the top and it feels firm to the touch, with just a bit of bounce.

To serve, invert the strainer to unmold the cheesecake onto a platter, remove the cheese-cloth, and slice into 8 wedges. Serve with the Balsamic Berries.

Balsamic Berries

½ pint strawberries
½ pint blackberries
½ pint raspberries
½ pint blueberries

4 tablespoons balsamic vinegar
4 tablespoons granulated sugar
½ cup dried cherries (see Note)
Pinch kosher salt

Wash all of the berries well in cold water and set aside to dry on paper towels. Hull the strawberries and slice them into quarters, then set them aside. In a large bowl, mix together the vinegar and sugar until the sugar dissolves. Add all of the fresh fruit and toss. Add the dried cherries and mix well. Let sit for at least 30 minutes before serving.

> **NOTE:** If the dried cherries are very tough, soak them for 30 minutes in warm water, then drain well before adding to the mix.

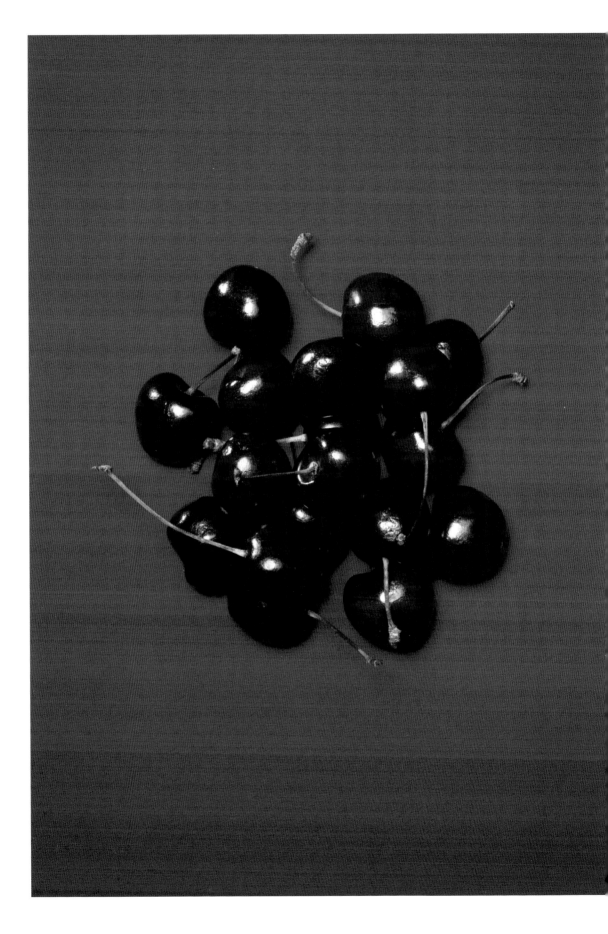

CHAPTER 2: Spiritual Wellness

SPIRITUAL WELLNESS IS ABOUT **BEING**. You've heard the expression, "Take time to stop and smell the roses." This really epitomizes the essence of what it means to do something that is spiritually healthful. More specifically, it means *being* several things. It's the difference between being mindful during everything you choose to do versus getting routinely distracted. It means being connected to something bigger than yourself, whether that's nature, religion, both, or something else entirely. Spiritual wellness is also about being in harmony with your community. For many, food shared within community is the ultimate spiritual connector.

COOKING for your spiritual well-being is about staying present and in the moment while you are preparing your meals. Instead of getting distracted and thinking of other things, you should focus only on what you are presently doing—stirring, slicing, spooning, etc. This does not mean laser focus on the specific task. Rather, it means getting lost in what things sound like, what they look like, and what they feel like. For example, while you are slicing vegetables, you should be thinking about the sound of the knife moving through each slice and along the cutting board; the sight of the rich, deep colors inside and outside each slice; the aromas that are released; and the textures, consistency, and temperature of the vegetables. The delicious recipes on the following pages give ample opportunity to stimulate your senses and truly enjoy cooking for yourself!

EATING for your spiritual well-being is about nurturing the communities within which you belong. Often, the perfect spiritual occasions are scheduled consistently throughout the year—birthdays, holidays, anniversaries, annual barbecues—but sometimes they come up unexpectedly, such as when a community member or family member deals with a health crisis or the loss of a loved one and the ensuing memorial services and gatherings. Use the recipes in this chapter to enjoy the perfect complementary foods for each of these occasions. But why wait for these dates to roll around to enrich your spiritual wellness through eating? Consider impromptu gatherings with your family, at work, and at play. Instead of "fitting them in," be sure to allow extra time so you can enjoy your meal and the people you've gathered together. Sharing these dishes with those closest to you is an excellent way to remain spiritually grounded and ensure that you are living in harmony with others. *The Self-Care Cookbook* is about taking time to "stop and smell the food," and the recipes in this chapter are no exception.

Spiritual wellness means being connected to something bigger than yourself—whether that's nature, religion, both, or something else entirely.

Tortellini Skewers with Brown Butter–Tomato Dip

SERVES 25 TO 30

This appetizer is great for gatherings and is a family favorite for potlucks. Food on a stick is fun for everyone, and you can vary the tortellini fillings or vegetables for your own palate. If there are leftovers, pull the pasta and veggies off of the skewers (along with any other chopped veggies from the veggie platter, if there was one) and toss with any leftover dip to create a wonderful pasta salad. The dip makes a terrific salad dressing as well.

2 pounds fresh tortellini of your choice
4–5 tablespoons extra virgin olive oil, divided
Kosher salt and freshly ground black pepper,
   to taste

3 (9-ounce) boxes frozen, quartered baby
   artichokes, thawed and patted dry
Brown Butter–Tomato Dip, for serving
   (recipe follows)

In a large pot of well-salted water, cook the tortellini according to the package directions. Drain and rinse under very cold water to stop the cooking—the tortellini should be cool to the touch. Transfer them to a large bowl, drizzle with 2 to 3 tablespoons of the oil, and toss to lightly coat. Add salt and pepper as needed. Set aside.

In a small bowl, toss the artichokes with the remaining 2 tablespoons of oil to lightly coat. Taste and add salt and pepper as needed.

To assemble, stick a tortellini on a small wooden skewer, followed by an artichoke quarter and then another tortellini. If you are using multicolored tortellini, try to use two different colors per skewer. Repeat this process until you've used all the tortellini.

Arrange the skewers on a platter with a bowl of the Brown Butter–Tomato Dip in the center. Serve chilled or at room temperature.

> **NOTE:** If you don't have time to make the dip, the skewers are also delicious with the store-bought pesto of your choice.
>
> I recommend the cheese-filled, multicolored tortellini because they're beautiful on the platter and are the easiest choice for the largest number of people. However, this recipe is equally delicious with meat or chicken tortellini!
>
> If you don't love artichokes, use small pieces of the vegetable of your choice; this is a great place to show your creativity. However, I don't recommend using canned or marinated artichokes here; the flavors are a little bit too aggressive.

Brown Butter–Tomato Dip

3 sticks unsalted butter
6 tablespoons sherry vinegar
6 tablespoons tomato sauce
2 tablespoons tomato paste
¾ cup extra virgin olive oil
2 tablespoons chopped shallot
2 teaspoons Dijon mustard
Pinch red pepper flakes (optional)
Kosher salt and freshly ground black pepper,
   to taste

In a small saucepan set over medium-high heat, melt the butter until browned but not burned, about 5 minutes. Remove from the heat and set aside, but be sure it does not congeal. To make the dip, the butter should be barely warm, but still liquid.

In a blender, combine the vinegar, tomato sauce and paste, oil, shallot, mustard, and red pepper flakes, if using. Blend until smooth. With the blender running, slowly drizzle in the butter and continue to blend until the dip has thickened. (You can also use an immersion blender.)

Taste and add salt and pepper as needed. Set the dip aside at room temperature until ready to serve. If you have to put it in the fridge, be sure to bring it back to room temperature before serving.

Salad-Bar Soup

SERVES 12

When you are cooking for community, especially in the case of sickness or bereavement, soup is one of the most soul-soothing things you can offer. Someone who is suffering physically or emotionally often can't bear the thought of many foods, but a simple hearty vegetable soup can go down easy. Making soup from scratch can often seem daunting, especially at scale, but this recipe uses salad-bar ingredients from the grocery store to lighten that load. This makes it an easy option when the need for soup is more immediate.

8 cups chopped assorted salad-bar vegetables
   (see Note)
1 (32-ounce) jar marinara or tomato–basil
   sauce of your choice
Pinch red pepper flakes (optional)
Kosher salt and freshly ground black pepper,
   to taste

1 large russet potato, peeled and cubed
½ cup dry small whole-wheat pasta, such as
   ditalini or orzo, or 8–16 ounces cooked
   plain salad-bar rice, pasta, or grains
¼ cup fresh flat-leaf parsley leaves, chopped

Dump the salad-bar vegetables into a large stockpot set over medium-high heat. Add the marinara and enough water (or good chicken or vegetable stock, if you have it on hand) to cover the vegetables by about 2 inches. Stir well and bring to a simmer.

When the soup is bubbling, add the red pepper flakes, if using, along with some salt and pepper. Add the potato and pasta. Cook for another 12 to 15 minutes, until the potato and pasta are cooked through. (If you are using cooked salad-bar rice, pasta, or grains, add them in for the last 5 minutes of cooking just to heat them through.) Add the parsley and stir well. Taste and add more salt and pepper as needed.

Serve hot or let cool before storing in the fridge for up to 5 days, or in the freezer for up to 3 months.

NOTE: The key to this soup is ease. You can use whatever raw veggies your local salad bar offers. Try shredded red cabbage, kale, carrots, celery, chickpeas, onion, zucchini, yellow squash, broccoli, or cauliflower—just make sure you use fairly equal proportions of each ingredient. (I don't like mushrooms in this soup; they make the broth sort of muddy.) You can also use any leftover cooked veggies you may have in the fridge. Add them in with the pasta and potato.

Asian Chicken Salad

SERVES 6 TO 8

This easy chicken salad is great for holiday luncheons or brunches. It's also the perfect thing to bring to a family managing a health crisis or a friend who's under the weather. If you want to start from scratch, use either the Classic Roast Chicken (page 71) or the chicken poaching technique from Poached Chicken with Broccoli Pesto (see page 16). Alternatively, grab a rotisserie chicken from the grocery store, remove the skin, and cube the meat. One whole chicken (or 3 large boneless, skinless breasts) provides the perfect amount for this recipe.

4 tablespoons granulated sugar

4 tablespoons unseasoned rice vinegar or white wine vinegar

2 teaspoons kosher salt

¼ teaspoon freshly ground white pepper

½ cup canola oil

1½ pounds cooked chicken, cubed

¼ cup toasted sesame seeds (see Note on page 159)

½ cup toasted almonds (see Note on page 159)

4 green onions, thinly sliced (including about 2 inches of the dark-green tops)

1 large head iceberg lettuce, cored and chopped, for serving

3½ ounces chow mein noodles or fried rice sticks, for garnish

To make the dressing, mix together the sugar and vinegar in a small bowl until the sugar dissolves. Add the salt and pepper. Slowly add the oil, whisking continuously until emulsified. Set aside.

Place the chicken, sesame seeds, almonds, and green onions in a gallon-size zip-top bag. Add the dressing, seal the bag, and smoosh around until everything is well coated and mixed. Transfer to the fridge to marinate for at least 4 hours or overnight. (The chicken can stay in the dressing for up to 3 days.)

To serve, arrange the lettuce in an even layer on a large platter. Add the marinated chicken, making sure to pour all of the dressing onto the chicken and lettuce. Garnish with the chow mein noodles and serve.

Roasted Lemon Shrimp with Pan-Fried Grit Cakes

SERVES 6 TO 8

Shrimp and grits don't always travel well, but this simple take on the Southern classic does, making them easy to add to a holiday buffet. You can also offer them to someone prepped, but not cooked, making them a good option to drop off to pals in need. Just prepare the shrimp on a baking tray and make the grit cakes, but don't do the final cook for either. You can deliver both trays, chilled, with simple cooking and reheating instructions.

3 pounds frozen cooked large shrimp
4 tablespoons unsalted butter, melted
½ teaspoon soy sauce
Zest of 1 lemon
2 tablespoons freshly squeezed lemon juice
½ teaspoon smoked paprika
½ teaspoon dried thyme

1 teaspoon kosher salt
½ teaspoon granulated sugar
¼ teaspoon freshly ground white pepper
Hot sauce, to taste (optional)
Pan-Fried Grit Cakes (recipe follows)
    or buttered rice, for serving

Preheat the oven to 400°F. Grease a baking sheet and set aside.

Thaw the shrimp under cold running water. Drain well and dry completely on a layer of paper towels, patting them down to get all the water off. Transfer the shrimp to a large bowl and set aside.

In a separate medium bowl, mix together the melted butter, soy sauce, lemon zest and juice, paprika, thyme, salt, sugar, pepper, and hot sauce, if using. Pour this mixture into the bowl of shrimp and toss until well coated.

Arrange the shrimp in single layer on the prepared baking sheet. Roast for 5 to 6 minutes, until the shrimp are hot. Serve over the Pan-Fried Grit Cakes.

> **NOTE:** I use frozen cooked shrimp here because they are easy to find and have already been prepped. If you are feeling ambitious, use fresh shrimp—just peel and devein them and extend the roasting time by 2 minutes.

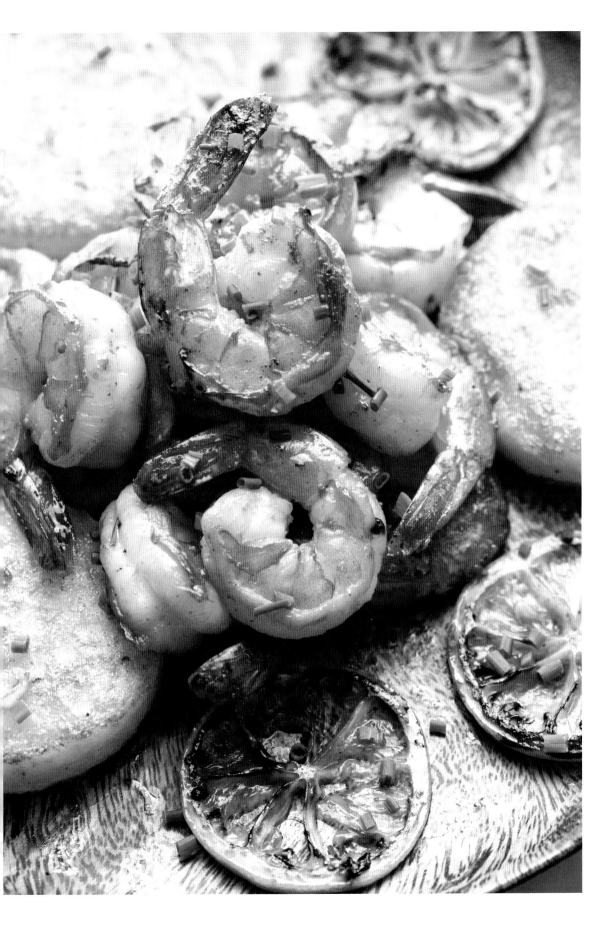

Pan-Fried Grit Cakes

2 cups water
1 teaspoon kosher salt
1 teaspoon freshly ground white pepper
4 tablespoons unsalted butter, divided
½ cup stone-ground grits

½ cup half and half
2 large eggs, beaten
1½ cups all-purpose flour, divided
2 tablespoons canola oil

Grease a 9 × 13-inch rimmed baking sheet and set aside.

In a medium saucepan set over medium-high heat, bring the water, salt, pepper, and 2 tablespoons of the butter to a boil. Add the grits in a slow stream, stirring constantly to avoid clumping, and cook, covered, for 5 to 6 minutes. Add the half and half, reduce the heat to medium low, and continue cooking, tasting and stirring frequently and adjusting the salt and pepper as needed, until the grits are tender but not mushy.

Transfer the cooked grits to the prepared baking sheet and store in the fridge for 2 to 3 hours, until firm. (Overnight is also fine; just cover them with plastic wrap if you plan on storing for longer than 2 hours.)

Flip the baking sheet over onto a cutting board. Cut the slab into 18 squares, then halve each slice diagonally, forming triangles.

In a shallow baking dish, place the beaten eggs. In a second shallow baking dish, place ½ cup of the flour, and place the remaining cup of flour into a third shallow baking dish. Line a large plate with paper towels and set the assembly line in the following order: dish with the least flour, dish with beaten eggs, dish with the most flour, plate.

Dip a grit cake in the smaller amount of flour and tap gently to get a thin coating. Next, dip the floured cake into the eggs, then dredge in the second dish of flour. Place the floured grit cake onto the prepared plate. Repeat until all the grit cakes have been covered.

Preheat the oven to 200°F. Grease another baking sheet and set aside.

Line another plate with paper towels and set near your stovetop. Heat the remaining 2 tablespoons of butter and the oil in a nonstick skillet set over medium-high heat. Add the grit cakes in batches and cook on both sides until golden brown and heated through. Once cooked, transfer the grit cakes to the prepared plate to drain.

After the grit cakes have drained, transfer them to the prepared baking sheet to make room on the plate. Once all the cakes have been fried and drained of oil, put the baking sheet in the oven to keep the cakes warm until ready to serve.

NOTE: You can also keep the cooked grit cakes at room temperature and reheat them in a 400°F oven for 10 minutes just before serving.

Parmesan Chicken Breasts

This is simple and can be easily multiplied, depending on how many people you are serving. It's also very versatile: kid friendly, buffet friendly, and an easy dinner for a family. Even if you serve it with a bag of frozen veggies and rice, you can get a balanced meal into someone who doesn't have the energy or ability to do it him- or herself.

4 (8-ounce) boneless, skinless chicken breasts
Kosher salt and freshly ground black pepper,
   to taste
1 large egg

¼ cup Dijon mustard
½ cup toasted breadcrumbs
½ cup grated Parmesan
4 teaspoons extra virgin olive oil

Preheat the oven to 400°F. Grease a rimmed baking sheet or roasting pan and place it in the oven to heat while you prepare the chicken.

Pat the chicken breasts dry with a paper towel and season well with salt and pepper. In a shallow bowl, mix together the egg and mustard until well blended. In another shallow bowl, mix together the breadcrumbs and Parmesan until well blended.

Dip a chicken breast in the egg mixture until well coated, let drip, and then dredge in the breadcrumb mixture, pressing it onto the chicken in an even layer. Set the breaded chicken aside on a plate and repeat this process with the remaining chicken breasts.

Carefully remove the baking sheet from the oven and place the chicken breasts on it in an even layer with space between them. Drizzle the top of each breast with 1 teaspoon of the oil. Bake for 15 to 18 minutes, until an instant-read thermometer inserted into the thickest part of the breasts registers 165°F.

Transfer the chicken to a plate and let rest for 10 minutes before serving.

NOTE: You can substitute 2 pounds of chicken tenders if you want to make this for an appetizer platter, but you might need to increase the breading amounts and reduce the cooking time by about half.

If you want to freeze this dish, let the chicken cool on the plate, uncovered, for 30 minutes instead of just 10, and then transfer them to a baking sheet in a single layer. Store in the freezer, uncovered, for 4 hours or overnight. Once frozen solid, you can put the chicken breasts in a zip-top bag. To reheat, preheat the oven to 400°F, place the frozen breasts on a greased baking sheet, and cook for 20 minutes, or until heated through.

Braised Brisket

SERVES 8

While this dish is often the centerpiece of traditional Jewish holiday dinners, this hearty, rich dish is a delicious addition to anyone's celebration. The leftovers make for amazing sandwiches and can be easily turned into pulled brisket or chili. It needs to be made at least a day before you want to serve it, but up to three days in advance is fine.

¼ cup water
1 (5-pound) beef brisket, trimmed but with a good layer of fat left on top
2 teaspoons kosher salt, plus more as needed
¼ teaspoon freshly ground black pepper, plus more as needed

2 large yellow onions, sliced
4 ribs celery, sliced
1 (12-ounce) bottle chili sauce, such as Heinz
1 (12-ounce) can beer (whatever you have around)
Balsamic vinegar, to taste (optional)

Preheat the oven to 350°F. Pour the water into a heavy roasting pan. Season the brisket with salt and pepper and lay it on top of the water. Spread the onions and celery over the top of the meat. Evenly add the chili sauce over the vegetables.

Roast, uncovered, for 90 minutes. Remove the pan from the oven, pour the beer over the meat and vegetables, cover the pan tightly with aluminum foil, and put it back in the oven to braise for 3 hours and 45 minutes, or 45 minutes per pound of meat. Remove the pan from the oven and let the meat rest for 30 minutes at room temperature.

Scrape the vegetables into a bowl and transfer the meat to a plate. Pour the gravy from the pan into an airtight container and let sit for 20 minutes to let the fat rise to the top. Transfer the container of gravy to the fridge for 20 to 40 minutes to let the fat solidify on top.

Remove the gravy from the fridge, then skim off and discard the fat. Transfer the gravy and vegetables to a blender and purée until smooth. Taste the gravy and add salt and pepper as needed. If the gravy needs brightness, add the balsamic vinegar, 1 teaspoon at a time, until the flavor is balanced. Transfer the gravy to an airtight container and wrap the meat tightly in plastic wrap. Chill both overnight in the fridge.

Remove the meat and gravy from the fridge. Slice the meat across the grain into ½-inch-thick slices and place them in a baking dish. Cover the slices with the gravy, cover the whole thing with plastic wrap, and store in the fridge for up to 3 days, or in the freezer for up to 2 months.

To reheat, remove the brisket from the fridge (if frozen, thaw the brisket in the fridge for 24 hours before reheating) and let sit at room temperature for at least 2 hours.

Preheat the oven to 350°F. Reheat, uncovered, for at least 1 hour. Once the dish is hot, reduce the oven temperature to 200°F, cover with foil, and keep it in the oven until ready to serve—almost indefinitely!

Slow-Roasted Pork Shoulder

SERVES 10 TO 12

This pork shoulder is the perfect centerpiece for any holiday gathering or large celebration. I first saw a version of this made by Jamie Oliver on one of his cooking shows and loved the idea. His version is a little fancier than mine, but this one eliminates some of the unnecessary fat. It is minimal effort, and since it cooks for about 10 hours in a low-temperature oven, it is very forgiving, allowing you to put your efforts and energies into spending quality time connecting to friends or family. As a bonus, it makes your house smell amazing!

2 tablespoons fennel seeds
1 teaspoon coriander seeds
1 teaspoon celery seeds
2 tablespoons kosher salt, plus more to taste
1 teaspoon ground Espelette pepper (optional)
½ teaspoon freshly ground black pepper,
   plus more to taste

1 (10–13-pound) pork shoulder on the bone,
   skin on
2 tablespoons grapeseed oil
2 cups water, plus more as needed
½ cup dry white wine
¼ cup apple butter

Preheat the oven to 500°F.

Heat a large skillet over medium heat until it feels warm but not uncomfortable when you place your palm a couple inches above its surface. Pour in the fennel, coriander, and celery seeds and toast, gently swirling the skillet to keep the spices moving, until they are slightly darker in color, have begun to glisten with released oils, and smell fragrant. Remove the skillet from the heat and transfer the toasted spices to a mortar. Add the salt, Espelette pepper, if using, and black pepper, and pound away with a pestle until you have a coarse, powdery mix. Set aside.

Score the pork shoulder skin about ¼ inch deep at 2-inch intervals all over, in two directions, making a nice diamond pattern. Rub the pork shoulder all over with the oil. Add the spice rub and work it into the pork skin in an even coat, making sure the rub is penetrating the score marks. Put the water into a large roasting pan and place the seasoned pork on top.

Roast, uncovered, for 30 minutes. Without opening the oven, reduce the oven temperature to 225°F and continue cooking for 9 to 11 hours, until the skin is very crispy and deeply browned and the meat pulls apart easily with a fork. Check periodically to ensure that there is a little liquid in the bottom of the pan, and add more water if it starts to dry out; you don't want the pan juices to burn or the pork to stick. Since every shoulder and every oven is different, start checking for doneness at the 8-hour mark.

CONTINUED ▷

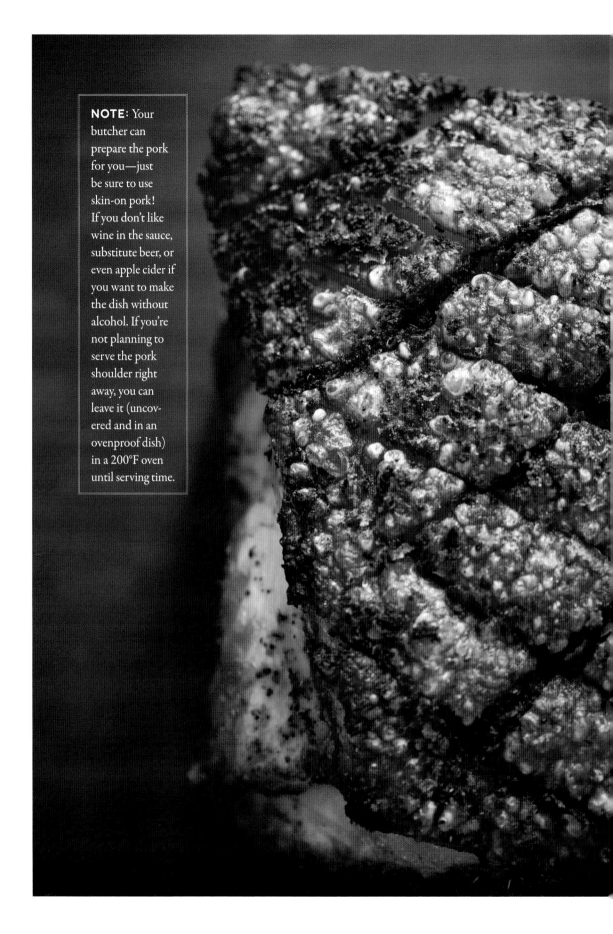

NOTE: Your butcher can prepare the pork for you—just be sure to use skin-on pork! If you don't like wine in the sauce, substitute beer, or even apple cider if you want to make the dish without alcohol. If you're not planning to serve the pork shoulder right away, you can leave it (uncovered and in an ovenproof dish) in a 200°F oven until serving time.

Slow-Roasted Pork Shoulder

CONTINUED

Remove the roasting pan from the oven and let the pork rest in the pan for at least 30 minutes. Transfer it to a large board or baking sheet. Pull off the cracklings in one large piece. Scrape any soft fat from the underside of the cracklings, remove any large pieces of fat from the surface of the meat, and discard the fat. Break the cracklings apart at the score lines or chop them into large pieces and set them aside.

Pour the pan juices into a small bowl and let sit for 10 minutes. Using a spoon, skim off the fat that has risen to the top. In a small saucepan, combine the juices with the white wine and cook over medium-high heat for 5 minutes to cook off the alcohol in the wine. Stir in the apple butter and continue to cook for 2 more minutes. Taste and add salt and pepper as needed. Remove the sauce from the heat and transfer to a serving bowl.

Using tongs or two forks, pull the meat apart into large pieces and arrange on a platter. Add the cracklings on the side and serve with a spoonful of the sauce.

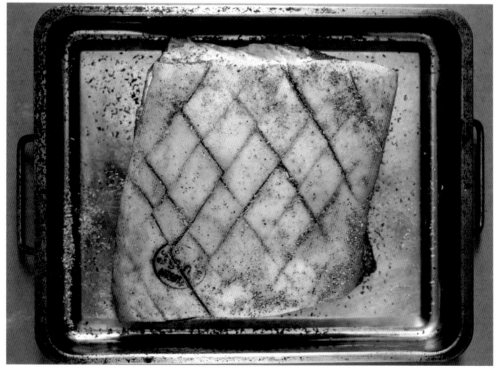

The seasoned and scored pork shoulder, ready for the oven.

Classic Holiday Turkey

SERVES 12 TO 14

I couldn't write a chapter about holiday and family gatherings without giving you a basic recipe for a perfect roast turkey, since it is the centerpiece of many holiday meals. This turkey works well for any large gathering. For a long time, I believed that wet brining was the standard for getting really moist turkey, but then I read a piece in the *Los Angeles Times* about dry brining. The premise is that if you wet brine, a lot of the newly introduced moisture is just water, which dilutes the turkey flavor. Dry brining, on the other hand, allows the meat to be fully seasoned and the juices are all the turkey's own. This revelation was a game changer. Dry brining is a terrific way to get a moist, flavorful bird that everyone around your table will love. It means you have to prep the turkey three days in advance, but I promise it is worth it!

3 tablespoons kosher salt, plus more to taste
1 tablespoon dried thyme
1 teaspoon sweet paprika
1 teaspoon freshly ground black pepper, plus more to taste
1 teaspoon minced fresh rosemary
Zest of 1 lemon
1 (12–16-pound) turkey, fresh or frozen and thawed

4 tablespoons clarified butter or ghee
4 large carrots, peeled
1 large onion, quartered
3 ribs celery
1 cup homemade or store-bought low-sodium chicken or turkey stock, or as needed
2 tablespoons chopped fresh herbs, such as thyme or marjoram (optional)

Three days before you want to cook the turkey, prepare the dry brine. In a small bowl, combine the salt, thyme, paprika, pepper, rosemary, and lemon zest, and mix well. Evenly coat the turkey with the dry brine and then put the turkey in a large zip-top brining bag. Press out as much air as possible and seal the bag. Place the bagged turkey on a baking sheet and transfer to the fridge. Once or twice a day, smoosh the turkey around in the bag.

The night before you cook the turkey, place a rack over a baking sheet, remove and discard the brining bag, and place the turkey on the rack. Return the turkey to the fridge, uncovered, and let it chill overnight. This dries the skin, which is the key to making it crispy!

The next day, remove the turkey from the fridge and leave at room temperature (uncovered) for at least 90 minutes.

Preheat the oven to 500°F. Rub the turkey all over with the clarified butter.

In a large roasting pan, place the carrots, onion, and celery in a single layer to create a bed for the turkey. Place the turkey, breast-side down, onto the vegetables.

Transfer to a rack in the lower third of the oven. Immediately reduce the oven temperature to 425°F and roast for 30 minutes. Remove the pan from the oven and carefully flip the turkey over so that the breast is facing up. The easiest way to do this is with wads of paper towels or a pair of clean dishcloths. If you are concerned, don't be afraid to enlist a friend to help!

Return the turkey to the oven and reduce the oven temperature to 325°F. Continue roasting for 2 hours to 2 hours and 45 minutes, until an instant-read thermometer inserted into the thickest part of the thigh (but not touching the bone) reads 165°F. Turkeys can vary widely, and so can oven temperatures, so start checking the bird's temperature after 90 minutes. Don't be afraid to pull it when the temperature is right; you definitely don't want it to overcook.

Transfer the turkey to a carving board. Let it rest, uncovered, for at least 30 to 40 minutes before carving. This may sound like a long time, but it will stay hot; this method guarantees juiciness.

To make the gravy, transfer the vegetables from the roasting pan to a blender. Pour the juices from the pan into a tall cup and set it aside for 10 minutes to allow the fat to rise to the surface. Skim off the fat, add the juices to the blender, and purée until smooth. If necessary, use the chicken stock to thin the gravy to your desired consistency. Taste and add salt and pepper as needed. Add the herbs, if using, for brightness. Transfer to a serving dish and set aside.

To carve, remove the leg and thigh quarters in a single unit, and then cut the leg from the thigh. At this point, the thigh will just have one bone in the center, which you can remove by making a slice right alongside the bone and gently pulling it away from the meat. The thigh meat can then be cut into 3 or 4 slices. Remove the 2 breast halves from the carcass whole, remove the wings, and then slice them across into ½-inch slices. Arrange the wings and legs in the center of a serving platter, then the dark meat on one half and the white meat on the other. Be sure to flip the bird over and get the two oysters, the tender nuggets of meat on either side of the backbone—they are the best cook's treat!

> **NOTE:** Ideally, you don't want a turkey that has been injected with juices—speak to your butcher about this!

Ravioli–Eggplant Lasagna

This is the perfect vegetarian dish for large gatherings and potlucks. I love to bring it to church picnics, block parties, and other celebratory events because it travels well and stays delicious even as it cools to room temperature. Vegetarians often feel as if their dietary needs take a back seat at big gatherings, so this dish will make them feel the love and satisfy the meat eaters of the group, too. This technique eliminates most of the fussy work involved with a traditional lasagna preparation, so you get all of the benefits of this classic Italian comfort dish with less than half the effort. By using store-bought frozen or fresh ravioli, you knock out the cheese and pasta layers in one fell swoop, so you can get lost in making the sauce and eggplant layers.

1 teaspoon kosher salt, plus more for sprinkling and to taste
2 large eggplants, cut into ½-inch-thick slices
3 tablespoons extra virgin olive oil, plus more for brushing
½ teaspoon freshly ground black pepper, plus more to taste
½ yellow onion, chopped
2 cloves garlic, minced
1 tablespoon tomato paste
1 teaspoon dried oregano

1 (15-ounce) can tomato sauce
1 (28-ounce) can whole peeled plum tomatoes (preferably San Marzano)
1 sprig fresh basil
Pinch red pepper flakes (optional)
2 (24–28-ounce) packages large, square cheese ravioli
1 cup grated Parmesan
1 cup shredded mozzarella
1 cup grated provolone

Preheat the oven to 450°F. Evenly grease 2 large baking sheets and then lightly sprinkle with salt. Place the eggplant slices on the prepared pans, brush the tops with oil, and season with salt and pepper.

Bake for about 6 minutes. Flip the eggplant slices over and continue cooking for 6 more minutes, or until the eggplant is tender and lightly browned. Set aside to cool.

In a saucepan set over medium-high heat, heat the 3 tablespoons of oil until it shimmers. Add the onion and cook until translucent, about 3 minutes. Add the garlic and cook for 1 minute. Add the tomato paste and oregano and cook, stirring frequently, for another 2 minutes. Add the tomato sauce and mix well.

Chop the canned tomatoes and add to the saucepan along with their juices. Add the basil, salt, pepper, and the red pepper flakes, if using. Reduce the heat to medium-low and simmer for 20 minutes. Taste and add salt and pepper as needed. Remove and discard the basil. Remove the sauce from the heat and set aside.

In a large pot, cook the ravioli in well-salted water for about half the time recommended on the package. You want the ravioli parcooked, just before it hits al dente, or it will get mushy later on. Meanwhile, in a small bowl mix together the Parmesan, mozzarella, and provolone. When the ravioli is parcooked, remove it from the heat and drain well, rinsing under cold water to stop the cooking.

Preheat the oven to 400°F and grease a 9 × 13-inch baking dish. To assemble the lasagna, place about one-third of the sauce in the dish in a thin layer. Add half of the cooked ravioli, arranging in a single layer. Then add half of the eggplant slices, trying not to overlap too much, in a single, solid layer. You may need to cut some of the slices to achieve this. Add another one-third of the sauce evenly on top, and then add half of the cheese. Repeat the layering process with the remaining half of the ravioli, the remaining half of the eggplant, the remaining one-third of the sauce, and the remaining half of the cheese. Depending on the size of your eggplant and ravioli, you may have a couple of extra pieces left over. This makes a great little snack or small lunch!

Bake for 12 to 15 minutes, until the lasagna is heated through and the cheese is golden and bubbling. Remove from the oven and let rest for 15 minutes. Slice and serve.

Confetti Rice Salad

SERVES 20 AS A SIDE

This vegan salad has no dairy and plenty of acid, so you can leave it on a buffet for hours without any concern about it going bad. It's delicious at room temperature and makes for a colorful addition to a potluck. It's gorgeous in a big bowl, but you can also stuff it into avocado halves or hollowed-out peppers or tomatoes for an elegant luncheon presentation.

Dressing
¼ cup freshly squeezed orange juice
¼ cup rice vinegar
¼ cup freshly squeezed lime juice
1 shallot, minced
1 tablespoon granulated sugar
1 teaspoon kosher salt
½ teaspoon freshly ground white pepper
1 tablespoon ground cumin
¾ cup canola or light olive oil

Salad
6 cups cooked white or brown rice, room temperature

1 (15-ounce) can black beans, rinsed and drained
⅓ cup diced celery
⅓ cup diced carrot
⅓ cup diced red bell pepper
⅓ cup cooked corn kernels, or canned baby corn sliced into rings
⅓ cup toasted pine nuts or almond slivers (see Note on page 159)
⅓ cup unpeeled diced green apple
⅓ cup very thinly sliced green onion (green and white parts)
⅓ cup fresh flat-leaf parsley leaves, chopped
Kosher salt and freshly ground black pepper, to taste

To make the dressing, in a small bowl whisk together all of the ingredients until emulsified. Taste and adjust the seasoning as needed. Set aside.

To make the salad, in a large bowl combine the rice, beans, celery, carrot, bell pepper, corn, pine nuts, apple, green onion, and parsley in a large bowl. Drizzle half of the dressing over the salad, mixing well with your clean hands (best way, trust me). Taste and continue adding the dressing as desired.

Reserve any leftover dressing; the salad may need it after it sits for a while. Taste and generously add salt and pepper as needed; items served cold or at room temperature often need more seasoning than hot dishes.

If serving the same day, let the salad sit at room temperature in a cool, dry place for at least 30 minutes and up to 4 hours to allow the flavors to meld and the rice to absorb the dressing. Taste and adjust the amount of dressing and seasoning as needed before serving.

> **NOTE:** After you cook the rice, do not cool it in the fridge. If the rice is cold, it will not absorb the dressing and will become tough.
>
> The diced ingredients should be small and uniform, about ¼ inch on each side.
>
> The dressed salad can be stored in the fridge in an airtight container for up to 1 week. Always let the salad come to room temperature for at least 1 hour before serving.

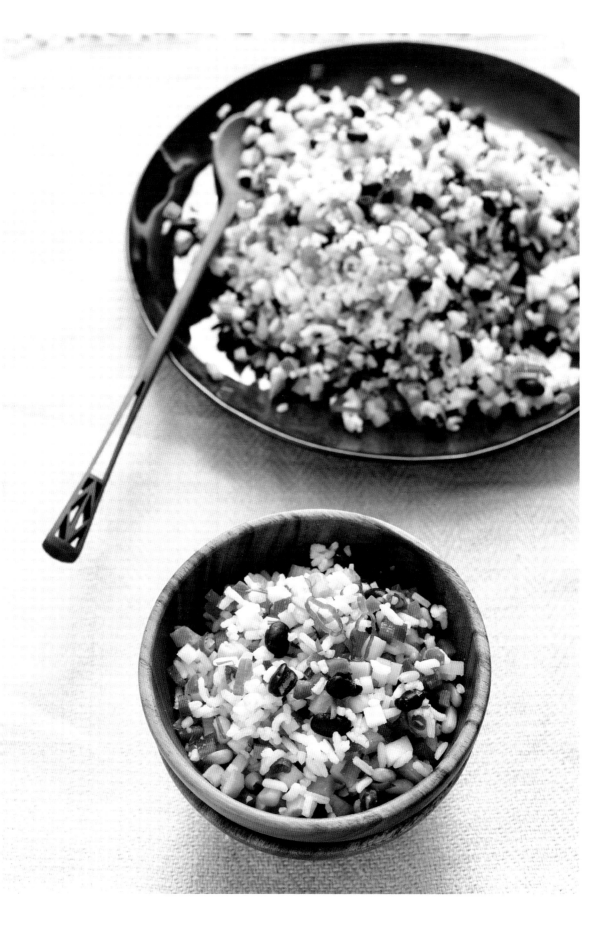

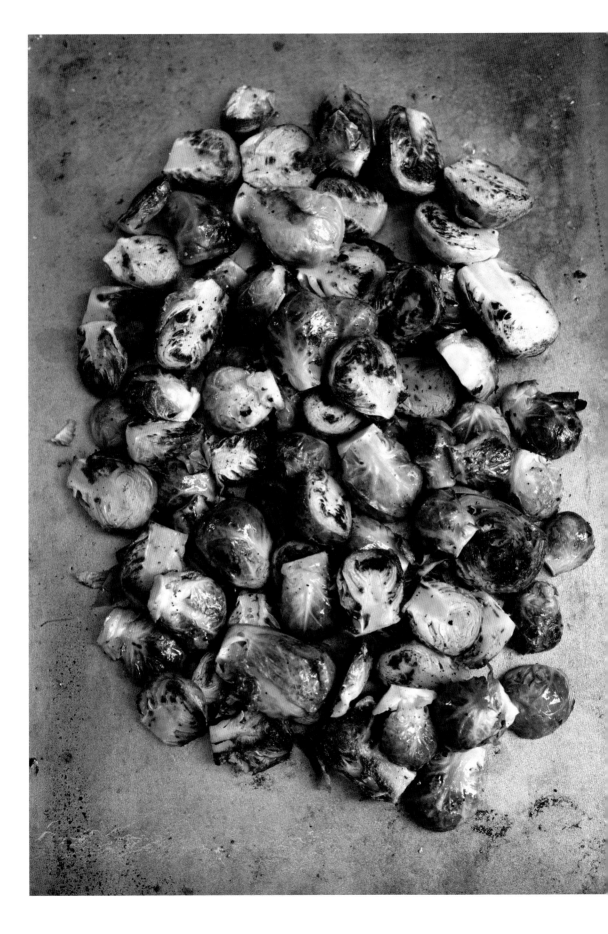

Caramelized Brussels Sprouts

Brussels sprouts are not often thought of as party food, and they're certainly not the typical thing you'd bring to someone in need of comfort. However, these crispy, caramelized beauties are absolutely delicious, and I can't tell you how many people I've converted to sprouts lovers with this easy side dish. There is something special about the connection you make with people when you make them fall in love with something they didn't think they liked at all. Plus, it's the perfect foil to the traditional meats we often see at holiday celebrations.

2 pounds fresh Brussels sprouts, trimmed and
   halved
3 tablespoons unsalted butter, melted

2 teaspoons granulated sugar
½ teaspoon kosher salt
¼ teaspoon freshly ground black pepper

Preheat the oven to 400°F. In a large bowl, toss together the sprouts and butter until well coated. In a separate small bowl, mix together the sugar, salt, and pepper. Add this mixture to the buttered sprouts and toss until they are all well coated.

Transfer the sprouts, cut-side down, to a baking sheet and roast for 15 minutes, until the outsides are browned and crispy and the insides are tender.

Remove from the oven, transfer to a serving bowl, and serve warm.

Wild Rice with Pistachios, Cherries, and Mint

SERVES 10 TO 12 AS A SIDE

One of the things I believe about spiritual cooking is that it can be a way to explore and appreciate other cultures—and to bring new and exciting flavors into the food you eat and serve to others. This simple pilaf is inspired by Mediterranean and Middle-Eastern flavor combinations, and presenting it in a group can open the conversation to other cultures in a positive way. This elegant side dish is a cinch to make, and the flavors are surprising. The fresh mint might seem odd, but the freshness it brings to the dish makes it a wonderful pairing with everything from chicken or pork to lamb or duck. You can play with the nut and fruit combinations; some of the ones I like are almonds and apricots, pine nuts and pomegranate seeds, hazelnuts and currants, and pecans and figs.

4 cups wild rice blend
½ cup red or white wine or apple juice
⅔ cup dried cherries
½ teaspoon ground cumin
4 tablespoons butter, melted

⅔ cup pistachios, chopped coarsely
4 tablespoons chopped fresh mint
2 tablespoons chopped fresh flat-leaf parsley
Kosher salt and freshly ground black pepper, to taste

Cook the rice according to package directions. While the rice is cooking, heat the wine and cherries in a small saucepan set over medium-low heat for 4 to 5 minutes, until the cherries plump. Remove the pan from the heat, discard the liquid, and set the cherries aside.

Once the rice is cooked, transfer it to a large serving bowl and fluff with a fork. You never want to use a spoon or spatula on rice or other grains; it will make them gummy. Set aside.

In a separate bowl, mix together the cumin and melted butter until well blended. Add the cumin butter, cherries, pistachios, mint, and parsley to the rice. Using two forks, mix the pilaf together. Taste and add salt and pepper as needed. Serve hot.

Peanut Butter Cup Brownies

MAKES 24

The only thing better than a brownie? A muffin-sized brownie with a chocolate chip cookie base and peanut butter cup in the middle. It's the perfect all-purpose offering, welcome whether you are bringing it to friends who are having a party or friends who are going through a tough time. They are both celebratory and comforting, and a terrific recipe to have in your back pocket.

3 squares unsweetened baking chocolate
2 sticks unsalted butter
4 eggs, beaten
2 cups granulated sugar
Pinch kosher salt
1 teaspoon pure vanilla extract

1 cup all-purpose flour
1 (16.5-ounce) package Nestlé Toll House chocolate chip cookie dough (use the mini cookie version, if available)
24 regular-size peanut butter cups, unwrapped

Preheat the oven to 350°F. Grease 2 (12-cup) nonstick muffin pans and set aside.

To make the brownie batter, melt the chocolate and butter together in a small saucepan over low heat, or in the microwave, and mix to blend well. In a separate large bowl, use a wooden spoon or rubber spatula to mix together the eggs, sugar, salt, and vanilla until well blended. Add the chocolate mixture and whisk to combine. Stir in the flour. Set the batter aside.

Into the prepared muffin pans, spoon about 1½ tablespoons of cookie dough (1½ cubes, if you're using the mini size) per cup and press into the bottom in an even layer. Add 1 peanut butter cup to each muffin cup. Pour in brownie batter so that each muffin cup is just shy of two-thirds full.

Bake for 15 to 18 minutes, until the brownies are firm. Remove from the oven and let the brownies cool in their pans for 5 minutes. Transfer the brownies to a wire rack to cool completely. Serve.

> **NOTE:** These treats are also great with mini peppermint patties or caramels in them. You can also make homemade cookie dough or try a peanut butter, sugar, or oatmeal cookie base.

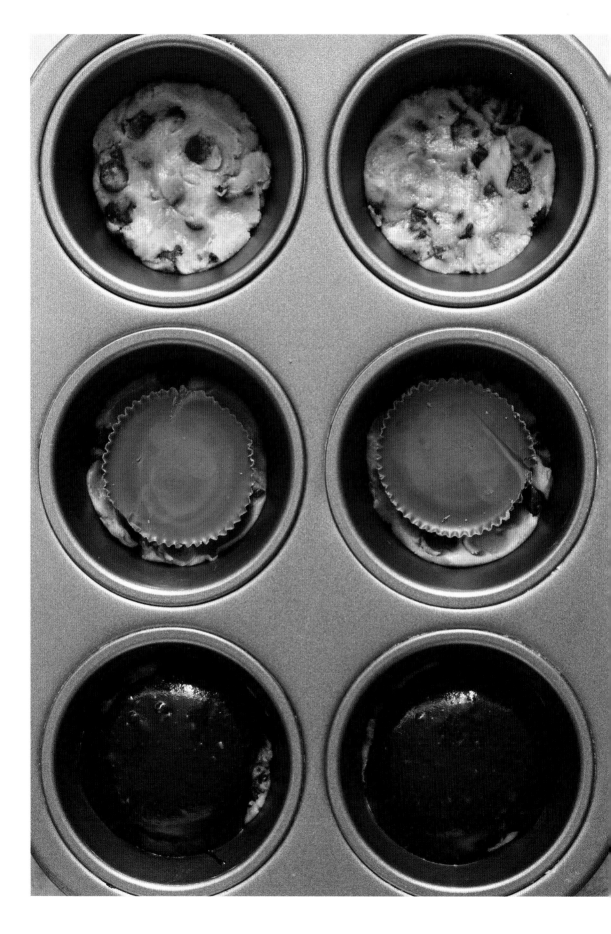

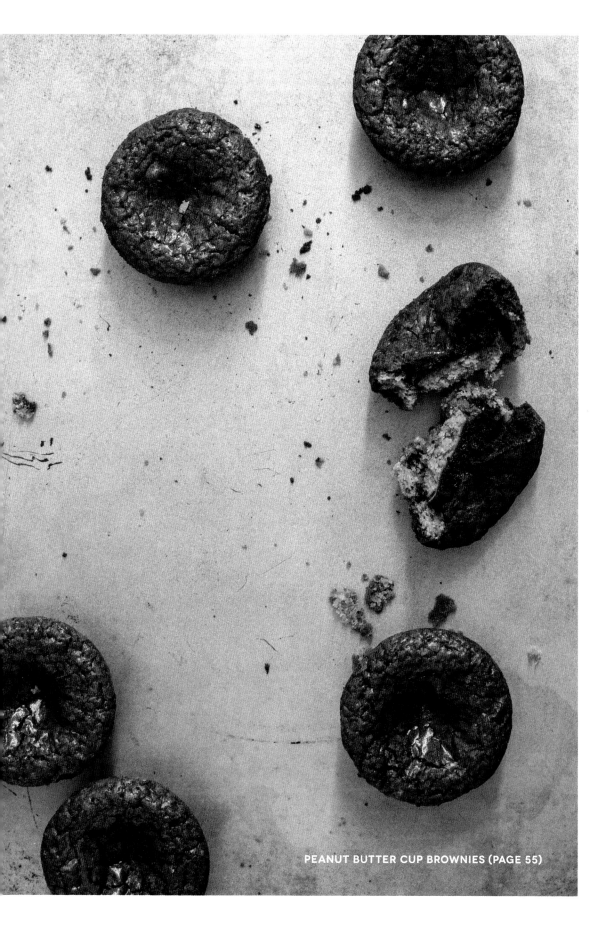

PEANUT BUTTER CUP BROWNIES (PAGE 55)

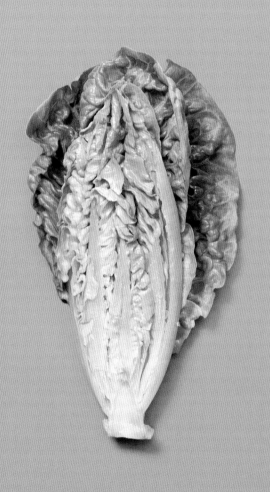

CHAPTER 3: Emotional Wellness

EMOTIONAL WELLNESS IS ABOUT **FEELING**. It includes being in touch with your emotions and what they mean. It is also about your ability to manage them, despite how turbulent life may be. The "common cold" of emotional health is stress—perhaps more accurately referred to as *distress*. Research suggests that stress is responsible for 70 percent of all disease and 40 percent of all deaths in the United States. Many stressors challenge us throughout our day, including traffic, relational discord, financial worries, and more. While we cannot always control these, we *can* choose to manage our feelings and our stress in a healthful way. One way to do this is to turn the time you spend cooking and eating into a relaxing, low-stress experience. Cooking thoughtfully and eating foods that bring comfort and joy are a way of supporting your emotional well-being. There is a reason that certain dishes are called "comfort foods," and knowing what those foods are for you and how to best embrace them as a part of your overall cooking and eating lifestyle can be a part of emotional wellness.

Turn the time you spend cooking and eating into a relaxing, low-stress experience.

COOKING for your emotional well-being means doing so in a manner that best manages negative life stressors. It also means cooking in a way that produces positive, affirming feelings. To make sure cooking doesn't accidently turn into another stressor, try "prepping for the prep" when you make the recipes in this chapter. Select your favorite music and a soothing beverage to enjoy while you make your meal. Adjust the lighting to a calming level. Silence your cell phone and reduce any other unnecessary distractors. Tell your loved ones that you are not to be disturbed unless it is absolutely necessary—make the kitchen your sanctuary. Finally, consider doing one full and slow diaphragmatic breath (from your stomach, not your chest) just prior to completing each step in your recipe. Now you can begin to cook in a stress-free way!

One final tip—be sure you give yourself extra time for food prep and take it nice and slow. If it normally takes you 15 minutes to pull together a particular recipe, allow time and a half, which in this example amounts to 20 to 25 minutes. Set the table, even if it's just for you. This is not the time to grab your meal in front of the television. Get out a nice plate, and plan on creating a nice-looking presentation of appropriate portions, the way a lovely restaurant would present it to you.

EATING for your emotional well-being means eating to nurture your feeling self. Everyone needs and can benefit from comfort, and the following recipes have been selected with your emotional well-being in mind—they are the epitome of comfort food. Select the ones that give you the most comfort and enjoy! While some will suggest that eating these foods is overly indulgent, I say this stems purely from a lack of understanding of what it means to be well. If you agree with the notion of "everything in moderation," then you should enjoy these scrumptious dishes accordingly. The serving sizes listed in these recipes represent a rational portion of each dish, allowing you to indulge thoughtfully.

Notice that nowhere in this chapter do I suggest that you pull into a fast-food drive-thru or grab a bag of chips. I suggest that, during times of emotional distress, you make a conscious choice to thoughtfully indulge in a food that has happiness properties. Foods like chocolate, nuts, strawberries, and others have chemical makeups that have been shown to impact the pleasure centers of the brain. And we often associate certain foods with good times or people we love, creating a happy memory when we eat them. Thoughtfully indulging in foods that make you happy, either chemically or through memory, can be a healthy part of your overall eating program. This may also ward off extra feelings of deprivation, feelings that can lead to overindulging in foods that are not as healthful for you later.

If you have used your prep time as I suggest, your stress should already be reduced by the time you get to the eating part, allowing you the opportunity to eat slowly and mindfully, and to fully enjoy every bite of a rational portion of your chosen indulgence. If you enjoy the occasional drink, this would be a time for a nice glass of the wine or beverage of choice that complements the foods you have chosen.

Edamame Dip

SERVES 8

Buddakan, a restaurant in New York City, serves edamame dumplings. There, these little pillows of perfection float in a Sauternes broth garnished with chive sprouts—the kind of dish that is deeply crave-worthy and wonderfully comforting. But let's be honest: when you want comfort food at home, you aren't going to start rolling dumpling dough or sourcing chive sprouts. When it comes to feel-good comfort foods, there is something oddly soothing about a dip. Dips, one of the first celebratory foods we learn to make as kids (i.e., mixing an onion soup packet into a tub of sour cream), almost always mean a gathering of friends or family, creating wonderful memories. This dip takes the essence of my favorite dumplings and turns them into something as easy as that onion dip. It works deliciously with crudités, but it is also a genius partner for potato chips or pita crisps, too.

3 cups cooked frozen shelled edamame, thawed
1 stick unsalted butter, softened
½ cup heavy cream
½ cup white truffle oil (see Note)

1 teaspoon kosher salt, plus more to taste
½ teaspoon freshly ground black pepper, plus more to taste
2 tablespoons chopped chives, for garnish

Bring a medium pot of salted water to a boil over medium-high heat and cook the edamame for 5 to 6 minutes, until they are super tender and mush easily under a spoon. Even though the edamame are fully cooked in the bag, they tend to be a bit al dente for this recipe; here you want total mush.

Drain the edamame well and transfer them to the bowl of a food processor or blender. Add the butter, cream, truffle oil, salt, and pepper and purée until smooth. Taste and add salt and pepper as needed.

Transfer to a serving bowl and garnish with the chives. Serve at room temperature.

> **NOTE:** Most truffle oils on the market don't actually have truffles in them, just chemical reproductions of truffle flavor, which is why you will hear chefs on television railing against their use. But, there are oils infused with actual truffles, and they are transcendent. Oregon Truffle Oil makes a good one. If you can't find real truffle oil, you can substitute a buttery olive oil or even almond oil, but you will lose some of the luxury of this recipe.

Butternut Squash and Pumpkin Soup

This soup can be served as a starter or as the main course of a meal. The mellow sweetness makes it feel like a treat, the velvety texture is amazing, and the variety of potential toppings means that it can be as rustic or refined as you choose. The most important thing is that it soothes the soul.

Soup
1 stick unsalted butter
2 medium yellow onions, diced
3 pounds peeled, cubed butternut squash
2 (29-ounce) cans pumpkin purée
　(not pumpkin pie filling!)
1 gallon homemade or store-bought low-
　sodium chicken stock or vegetable stock,
　or water, divided

1 pint heavy cream
¼ teaspoon ground nutmeg
¼ teaspoon ground Espelette pepper (optional)
Kosher salt and freshly ground white pepper,
　to taste

Topping
½ cup cold heavy cream
8–10 amaretti cookies, crumbled

Place a medium metal bowl in the freezer for at least 1 hour.

To make the soup, melt the butter in a large stockpot set over medium-high heat until the foaming subsides. Add the onions and sauté until they are soft and translucent. Add the squash and pumpkin purée. Add enough of the chicken stock to cover by about 2 inches, and set the rest aside.

Give the pot a good stir. Bring the mixture to a simmer, reduce the heat to medium, and cook, uncovered, until the squash is very soft, 35 to 45 minutes. If it begins to boil, reduce the heat to low; you want it at a simmer.

Remove the soup from the heat and let cool for at least 1 hour. Using an immersion blender, blend the soup in the pot (or in batches in a regular blender) until very smooth. For extra-velvety soup, strain through a chinois or fine-mesh strainer.

Bring the soup back to a simmer over medium heat. Add the cream, nutmeg, and Espelette pepper, if using. Taste and add salt and white pepper as needed. Using white pepper here is more of an aesthetic choice, since the soup is prettier without black pepper flakes in it, but it isn't essential if all you have is black pepper. If the soup is too thick, add the reserved chicken stock until you get a texture you like. Keep the soup at a simmer until ready to serve.

CONTINUED ▷

Butternut Squash and Pumpkin Soup
CONTINUED

To make the topping, pour the cream into the chilled metal bowl. Using an electric handheld mixer set on medium speed, whip the cream just until stiff peaks form. Add the crumbled amaretti cookies and stir gently until combined.

To serve, portion the soup into bowls and garnish with a dollop of the topping. Serve right away.

ALTERNATIVE TOPPINGS

- Crushed gingersnaps
- Crème fraîche mixed with crystallized ginger
- Candied orange zest
- Toasted gingerbread croutons
- Caramel corn
- Whipped cream blended with cranberry sauce
- Croutons with melted Asiago
- Fried sage leaves
- Crispy bacon or pancetta
- Diced pear or apple
- Cinnamon sour cream
- Toasted pumpkin seeds

NOTE: This soup freezes beautifully, but you need to freeze it before adding the cream, and adjust seasonings once you have added the cream the day you serve. This recipe makes a large batch, suitable for holiday meals, but if you want it for a smaller gathering, you can freeze half and add cream only to the portion you are serving that day. You can keep this soup up to 3 days in the fridge, but I recommend adding the cream and seasonings the day you serve it.

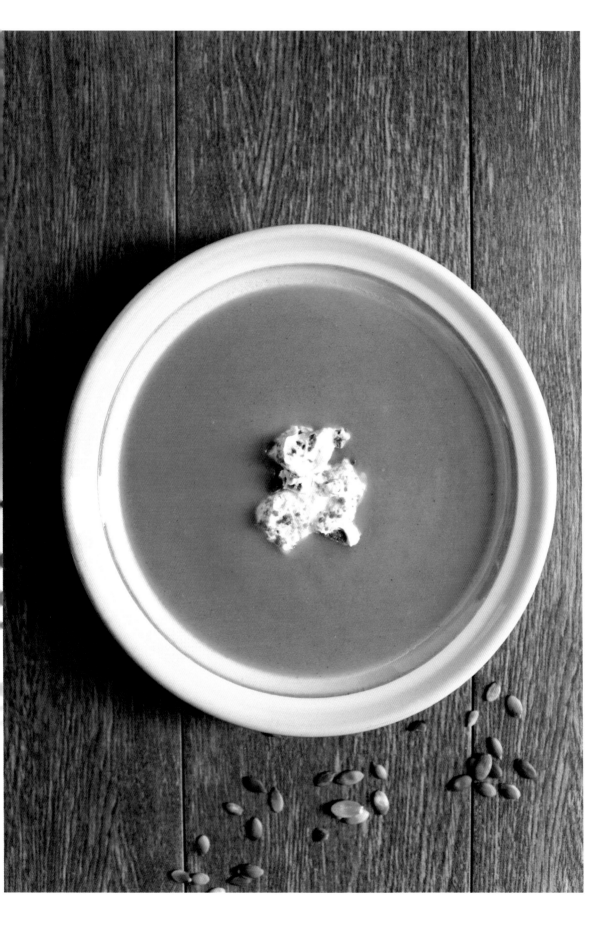

Classic Wedge Salad

SERVES 4

One of the reasons that most comfort foods are also old classics is because the flavors remind us of a past happy time. Many people have forgotten how wonderful a crisp wedge of Thousand Island–topped iceberg lettuce can be. Bottled Thousand Island dressings tend to be claggy and overly sweet, turning many people off. This homemade dressing is bright and balanced, and the sweet and crunchy lettuce is the perfect foil. I've added even more happy-inducing elements with roasted grape tomatoes and crispy nuggets of bacon, but the salad is terrific without either. The dressing also works well as a dip.

1 pint grape tomatoes or small cherry tomatoes
1 tablespoon canola or grapeseed oil
½ teaspoon granulated sugar
¼ teaspoon kosher salt
8 ounces thick-sliced bacon

1 large head iceberg lettuce
  (see Note on page 67)
1 recipe Thousand Island Dressing (recipe
  follows)
Freshly ground black pepper, to taste
2 tablespoons chopped chives, for garnish

Preheat the oven to 400°F. In a small roasting dish, toss the tomatoes with the oil, sugar, and salt. On a baking sheet, arrange the bacon in a single, even layer.

Transfer the bacon to the upper rack of the oven and the tomatoes to the bottom rack. Roast for 15 to 20 minutes, until the bacon is very crisp and the tomatoes have begun to wrinkle. Remove from the oven. Set the tomatoes aside to cool in their dish, and transfer the bacon to a paper-towel-lined plate to drain. Once the bacon has cooled, cut it into strips.

Core the lettuce and remove and discard any limp outer leaves. Cut it into 4 wedges and arrange them on plates.

To assemble the salad, top each wedge with a generous spoonful of the Thousand Island Dressing. Add the sliced bacon and roasted tomatoes and season generously with pepper. Garnish with the chives. Serve the wedges with any extra dressing on the side.

Thousand Island Dressing

1 cup good-quality mayonnaise, like Hellmann's
½ cup Heinz chili sauce
2 tablespoons sour cream
1 teaspoon freshly squeezed lemon juice
1 tablespoon sweet pickle relish
2 tablespoons finely chopped celery hearts
1 teaspoon Worcestershire sauce
Pinch red pepper flakes (optional)
Kosher salt and freshly ground black pepper,
    to taste

In a small bowl, thoroughly combine the mayonnaise, chili sauce, sour cream, lemon juice, relish, celery hearts, Worcestershire sauce, and red pepper flakes, if using. Taste and add salt and pepper as needed. Transfer the dressing to an airtight container and store in the fridge for up to 1 day or until ready to use.

> **NOTE**: When choosing iceberg lettuce, look for a head that feels heavy for its size and is free of brown or mushy spots. The stem should not look slimy. When making the dressing, avoid Miracle Whip; it will be too sweet.

Lobster Tails with Herb–Butter Sauce

SERVES 2

Sometimes the best way to give yourself an emotional boost is to prepare and eat something that feels luxurious and decadent, a special treat. I associate those special foods with special occasions and happy celebrations, and bringing those foods into my eating life during times of stress or emotional strain can be a real mood booster. This is an elegant dish with a luxurious punch that is surprisingly easy to make. While whole lobsters can be fun, they are something of a messy and complicated endeavor, and the point of this meal is connecting over wonderful food, not engaging in a deconstruction project! Serve this with simple sides, like rice and steamed snap peas, both of which soak up the buttery sauce brilliantly.

1 teaspoon canola oil
1 small shallot, finely minced
¼ cup dry white wine or vermouth
½ cup lobster stock or fish stock
4 tablespoons unsalted butter, cut into
   1-tablespoon chunks and chilled
½ cup water

½ tablespoon minced fresh tarragon
1 tablespoon minced fresh flat-leaf parsley
1 tablespoon chopped chives
Kosher salt and freshly ground white pepper,
   to taste
2 (8-ounce) large raw lobster tails, shells on

Bring a large pot of well-salted water to a boil over medium-high heat.

Meanwhile, in a medium sauté pan set over medium-high heat, heat the oil until it shimmers. Add the shallot and cook for about 2 minutes, until it is translucent. Reduce the heat to medium-low and add the wine. Cook, stirring occasionally, until the wine is reduced to a glaze on the bottom of the pan, 3 to 4 minutes. Stir in the stock and bring to a simmer.

Add the cold butter very slowly, 1 piece at a time, whisking until the butter is fully blended before adding the next piece. You are creating a beurre monté, a sauce made of butter that has been mixed with a liquid to create a smooth emulsion. It's not hard; it just requires precision. Continue this process until all the butter is fully incorporated. Keep a close eye on the heat and reduce it if it looks like the mixture might start to boil; boiling will make the butter separate.

Add the tarragon, parsley, and chives. Taste and add salt and pepper as needed. Cover and reduce the heat to low.

At this point, the water should be boiling. Add the lobster tails and boil for 4 to 5 minutes, until the shells of the lobster tails are bright red and have curled up a bit on themselves. Remove them from the water and let rest for 4 minutes.

Using a pair of kitchen shears, cut a slit up the underside of the tails and remove the meat. Discard the shells. The lobster meat should be pink on the outside, opaquely white on the inside, and slightly firm when gently touched with your finger. It should not feel mushy, rubbery, or bouncy.

Transfer the cooked tails to a cutting board and slice into ½-inch-thick pieces. Fan the lobster slices on plates in a pretty half-moon shape. Remove the sauce from the heat and generously spoon over the slices. Serve right away.

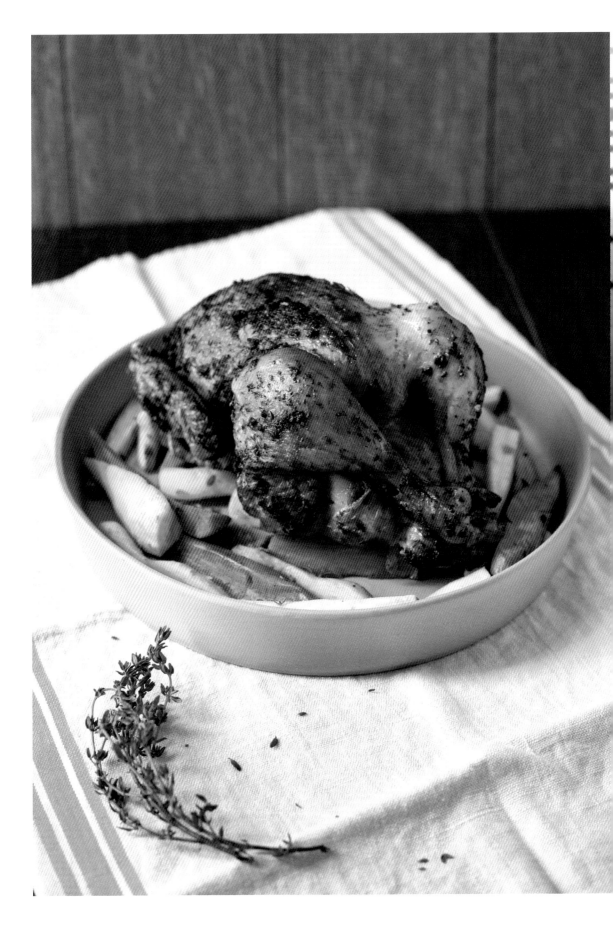

Classic Roast Chicken

SERVES 4

Sometimes, when we need emotional grounding, what we need is simplicity. There is nothing more basic than a roasted chicken. It fills the house with a soothing smell, and the flavor is simple but deeply satisfying. While many recipes for roast chicken involve all sorts of seasonings or rubs, flavored butters under the skin, or aromatics stuffed in the cavities, this one does not. This recipe embraces the idea that sometimes, what we need most is the least complicated.

1 (3-pound) organic whole chicken
1 tablespoon canola or grapeseed oil

1 tablespoon kosher salt, plus more as needed
Freshly ground black pepper, to taste

Preheat the oven to 450°F.

Remove and discard the giblets bag, if there is one, from the chicken. Pat the chicken dry all over with paper towels; you want the chicken as dry as possible so that the skin will crisp nicely.

Rub the outside of the chicken with the oil. Coat the chicken all over with the salt. The best way to do this (or to season any meat) is to take a pinch of the salt between your thumb and first and middle fingers, hold your hand at about eye height over the meat, and let the salt rain down evenly. This allows the salt to disperse uniformly, and you can avoid having patches of oversalted or undersalted meat. Use your other hand to turn the chicken as you sprinkle. Use more salt if you run out before you cover the whole bird.

Place the seasoned chicken in a roasting pan and transfer to the oven. Roast for 50 minutes to 1 hour, until an instant-read thermometer inserted into the thickest part of the thigh registers 165°F. While the chicken cooks, set a wire rack over a shallow pan and set close to the oven.

When the chicken is done, transfer it to the prepared wire rack. Let the bird rest, uncovered, for 20 minutes. Resting is key here: the chicken will finish cooking during this time, and the temperature may rise as much as 5°F to 10°F. More important, resting allows the meat to relax and reabsorb all of its juices. If your meats or poultry leave large puddles of juice on your cutting board, you have cut them too soon—rest them longer next time!

To carve, transfer the chicken to a cutting board. Remove the legs and thighs in one piece, and then separate the thigh from the leg, if desired. Cut the breast meat off the bone with the wings still attached. Cut the breast into two pieces, one the wing with a large piece of breast meat and one the rest of the breast. Transfer to a platter and serve.

Pork Schnitzel

SERVES 6

Nothing is quite as satisfying as something with a crispy, crunchy, fried exterior. And the act of breading the schnitzel can be a little bit meditative, which can help you de-stress. When I started this project Stacey recommended that I start to pull recipes from cooking magazines so that we could use them as inspiration. When I saw a version of this in *Food and Wine* magazine I knew I wanted to see if we could incorporate it into this book, since I lived in Wisconsin for a while and always appreciated the German food I had there. If you don't want to do this with pork, it is equally fantastic with chicken or veal. Schnitzel is a quick, delicious dinner and pairs well with something bright and acidic, like a German-style potato salad; mixed greens with a Dijon vinai-grette; or even white beans dressed with oil, vinegar, and a lot of parsley. Leftovers make terrific sandwiches, which is why this recipe serves six—yes, it will be great for a small dinner party, but it will also serve four with some leftovers!

1⅓ cups all-purpose flour
3 large eggs, beaten
3 tablespoons water
3 cups plain breadcrumbs
Kosher salt and freshly ground black pepper,
   to taste

6 (4–5-ounce) boneless pork cutlets, pounded
   to ⅓ inch thick
Grapeseed oil, for frying
1 lemon, quartered, for serving

Make a classic breading station by setting out 3 shallow rectangular baking dishes. In the first dish, put the flour. In the second, put the eggs and water, mixing them well. In the third, put the breadcrumbs. Add a large pinch of salt to both the flour and the breadcrumbs and mix with a fork until the salt is incorporated. Set a lightly greased rack on a baking sheet and place it next to the breading station.

Season both sides of the pork cutlets with salt and pepper.

With your right hand, dip a cutlet into the flour and flip it a couple of times, coating on all sides. Shake it gently to remove any excess; you are looking for a light dusting of the flour, which will help the egg stick, which will make the breadcrumbs stick. If you skip this step, your coating will likely slide off the cutlets when you cook them.

Slide the floured cutlet into the egg mixture to coat and then flip it with your left hand to get a good coating, keeping your right hand dry. Transfer the cutlet to the bread-crumbs. Again with your right hand, sprinkle the breadcrumbs on top of the cutlet, press a bit, and flip the cutlet over until well coated. Give the cutlet a good pressing at the end to make sure the breadcrumbs are stuck on. Set the breaded cutlet on the pre-pared rack and repeat the process with the remaining cutlets.

Line a tray with paper towels and set it near your stovetop. In a large high-sided skillet set over high heat, heat about ½ inch of the oil until it shimmers. Reduce the heat to medium-high. Add 2 or 3 of the breaded pork cutlets in a single layer and cook, turning once, for 3 to 4 minutes, until golden and crispy. Transfer the schnitzel to the prepared tray, season with a bit more of the salt, and let drain. Repeat this process with the remaining cutlets. If necessary, you can keep the cooked schnitzel warm in a 200°F oven, on a rack over a baking tray.

Serve the schnitzel hot with the wedges of lemon.

NOTE: When setting up a breading station, a lot of people use bowls, but I prefer to use the baking dishes specified in this recipe. Their shape makes it easier to handle and manipulate ingredients. When coating anything with this setup, it's best to keep one hand dry and one hand wet.

Grilled-Cheese Cheeseburgers

SERVES 4

When it comes to comfort-food sandwiches, grilled cheese and cheeseburgers are often favorites. In this perfect mash-up, very thin grilled-cheese sandwiches serve as both the bun and cheese component for your burger! They are a fun, delicious twist and great to make with kids, especially if they are feeling down about something. They are sort of silly and fun, and connecting over cooking can be very positive for all involved.

1 pound ground beef
Kosher salt and freshly ground black pepper, to taste
4 tablespoons unsalted butter, very soft

8 slices Pepperidge Farm Very Thin White Bread
4 slices American cheese

Preheat the oven to 200°F. Line a small baking sheet with paper towels or parchment paper and set aside. Set a wire rack over a shallow pan and set aside.

Divide the beef into 4 equal pieces and form into patties roughly the same size and shape as the bread slices. Season the beef well on both sides with salt and pepper.

Butter one side of each of the bread slices. The butter needs to be completely soft or you will never manage. With the buttered sides of the bread facing outward, make 4 cheese sandwiches (1 cheese slice per sandwich).

Set a large nonstick skillet or griddle over medium-high heat. Test for heat by holding your hand over the pan about an inch and a half from the surface; you should feel strong heat radiating from the surface and should not be able to hold your hand there very long. Transfer the sandwiches to the skillet and cook for about 90 seconds, or until the bottom slice is golden brown and crispy. Use a spatula to peek underneath. Carefully flip the sandwiches over and brown well on the other side. Transfer to the prepared baking sheet and keep the sandwiches in the oven while you cook the burgers.

Using the same skillet, increase the heat to high and cook the patties for 2 minutes per side, or until each side develops a browned crust. Then continue to cook to your preferred doneness. Transfer the burgers to the prepared wire rack and let them rest for 10 minutes.

Remove the grilled-cheese sandwiches from the oven. To assemble, place 1 burger patty between 2 sandwiches. Serve right away.

> **NOTE**: If you want to go a step further, you can also enhance the grilled cheese by adding crispy cooked bacon, caramelized onions, or a slice of ripe tomato before cooking. Add whatever garnishes you like!

Rack of Lamb with Mint–Pistachio Pesto

SERVES 2

Emotional wellness means being open about your emotions with the ones you are closest to, and that means having moments of quiet connection to express those emotions
one-on-one, whether it is a complicated conversation or just a moment of offering
appreciation for what the other person means to you. A lovely, elegant dinner for two
offers the opportunity to have those deeper communications. Rack of lamb feels like
special-occasion food, but it's easy to make. And while I still hold a fondness and nostal-
gia for the traditional mint jelly of my youth, I think this mint pesto is a much more
elegant way to go. The pesto is a great twist on an old favorite, and it is a fun recipe
to have in your repertoire; it works well with chicken or pork, or it can be an exciting
garnish for vegetables or pasta.

1 rack (8–9 ribs) lamb, frenched (your butcher
   can do this for you)
Kosher salt and freshly ground black pepper,
   to taste

1 tablespoon grapeseed oil
1 recipe Mint–Pistachio Pesto (recipe follows)

Preheat the oven to 450°F.

Season the lamb all over with the salt and pepper. In a large ovenproof skillet set over
high heat, heat the grapeseed oil until it shimmers. Add the lamb, fat-side down, and
cook for 2 to 3 minutes, until a brown crust forms. Flip the rack over, so that the ribs
curve downward, and transfer the skillet to the oven.

For rare, roast the lamb for about 15 minutes, until an instant-read thermometer stuck
sideways into the center of the eye of the meat registers 125°F. For medium rare, roast
the lamb for about 18 minutes, until the thermometer registers 130°F. Start checking
for doneness after 13 minutes. While the lamb roasts, place a wire rack over a pan and
set near the oven.

Carefully remove the skillet from the oven, transfer the lamb to the prepared wire rack,
and let rest for 15 minutes. Carve the ribs and serve right away with the Mint–Pistachio
Pesto on the side.

> **NOTE**: As always, be sure to have an oven mitt nearby—you'd be surprised how strangely
> instinctive it is to just grab the skillet handle when it is time to remove the lamb from the oven!
> A good tip is to keep an oven mitt draped over the handle of the oven to remind you.

Mint–Pistachio Pesto

3 cups lightly packed fresh mint leaves
¼ cup shelled toasted pistachios (see Note on
    page 159)
1 clove garlic
½ cup extra virgin olive oil, divided
Kosher salt and freshly ground black pepper,
    to taste

In a blender or food processor, pulse the mint, pistachios, garlic, and ¼ cup of the oil until a coarse paste forms. With the machine running, drizzle in the remaining ¼ cup of oil until the mixture is thick and creamy. Be sure to stop the blender as soon as you see the consistency you want, as overprocessing can make the oil bitter. Taste and add salt and pepper as needed.

Transfer the pesto to an airtight container and store in the fridge until you are ready to serve, up to 1 week. If you don't serve the pesto right away, spoon a thin layer of oil over the top before refrigerating to prevent browning.

Stewed White Beans with Tomatoes and Sage

SERVES 4 AS A SIDE

I think of this dish as vegetarian comfort food; it's soothing, filling, and good for the body and spirit. It is a great dish to have in your back pocket for when those unexpected stressors rear their heads, whether it is a lousy day at work for you or your partner, a child who has a rough day at school, or a friend or loved one who calls with their own issues. It comes together very quickly, so it becomes a good option for a last-minute dish, when you or someone close to you is in need of some immediate emotional support. If you make this as an entrée, I recommend serving over buttered rice, with a poached egg on top for even more protein.

2 tablespoons extra virgin olive oil or garlic oil

2 (15-ounce) cans cannellini beans (or any white bean), drained and rinsed

1–2 ripe tomatoes, cored and seeded, or 1 (15-ounce) can whole plum tomatoes, drained and chopped

6 fresh sage or basil leaves, chopped

Kosher salt and freshly ground black pepper, to taste

In a large skillet set over medium-high heat, heat the oil until it shimmers. Add the beans and tomatoes and sauté until melded and heated through, about 10 minutes. Stir in the sage and taste and add salt and pepper as needed. Continue to cook for 5 to 10 minutes more, until some of the beans break down a bit and combine with the oil and tomatoes to make a sort of sauce.

Remove from the heat. Serve hot or at room temperature.

> **NOTE:** If you do not have store-bought garlic-flavored oil, you can add two lightly crushed garlic cloves to the olive oil as you are heating it, and, once the cloves are golden brown, discard them. This will give you a lightly-scented garlic oil that will enhance, but not overwhelm, the delicate flavor of the beans. It is a good way to add mild garlic flavor to any recipe where you want a perfume of garlic and not a powerful punch!

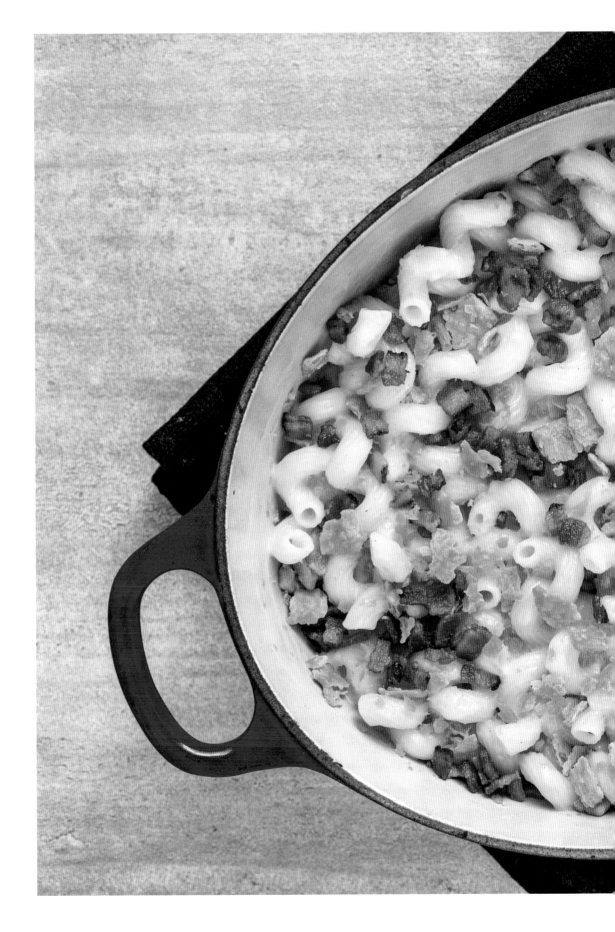

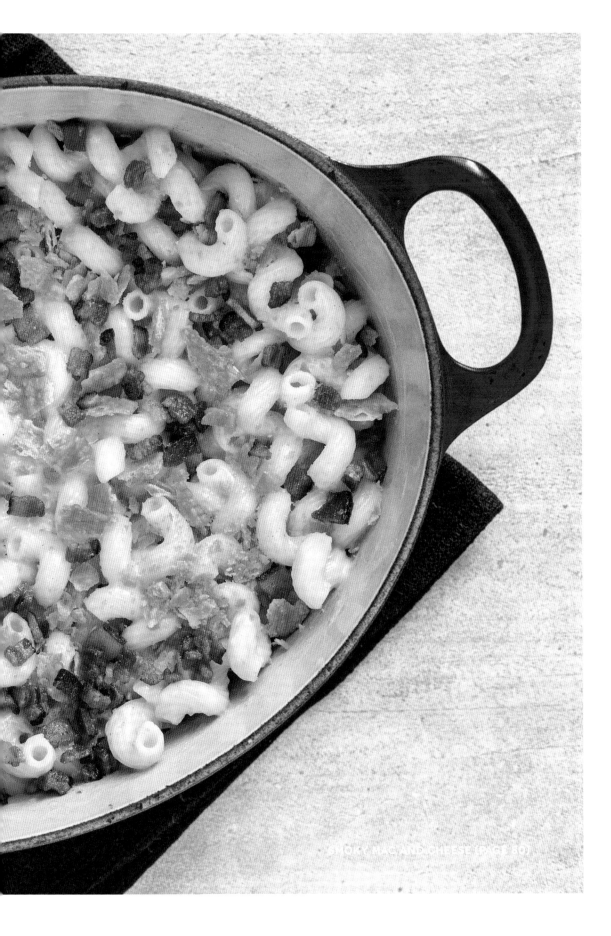

SMOKY MAC AND CHEESE (PAGE 80)

Smoky Mac and Cheese

I'm pretty sure I don't need to tell you the emotional benefits of a bowl of creamy macaroni and cheese. While the frozen brick and the blue box have their places, I strongly encourage you to give this homemade version a try. Pasta has two different chemicals that help release endorphins, which is why so many of us crave various noodle-based dishes when we need mood boosting. This slightly smoky version of the classic is very grown up and a terrific side dish for a party, but it also has enough of the flavors you remember from your childhood to be everything you want it to be in terms of comfort. The Cheez-It topping brings in an element that is fun and surprising, and nothing is more soul soothing than bacon!

1 pound cavatappi, gemelli, or elbow macaroni
5 tablespoons unsalted butter
6 tablespoons all-purpose flour
1 tablespoon mustard powder
½ teaspoon grated nutmeg
½ teaspoon smoked paprika
5 cups whole milk
8 ounces fontina, grated
4 ounces smoked Gouda, grated

8 ounces extra-sharp white Cheddar, grated
½ cup sour cream
Kosher salt and freshly ground black pepper, to taste
½ cup crumbled Cheez-It crackers
3 tablespoons melted unsalted butter
4 slices extra-thick bacon, cooked until crisp and crumbled

Preheat the broiler. Grease a 9 × 13-inch baking dish and set aside.

In a large pot of well-salted water, cook the pasta according to the package directions until just shy of al dente. Reserve 1 cup of the pasta water and set aside. Drain the cooked pasta and set aside.

While the pasta is cooking, melt the butter in a large saucepan set over medium-high heat until the foaming subsides. Sprinkle the flour evenly over the melted butter and whisk to combine. Cook, whisking constantly, for 2 minutes. Add the mustard, nutmeg, and paprika, and continue to whisk constantly for 1 minute. Briskly whisk in the milk to combine and cook, still whisking constantly, for about 5 minutes, or until the mixture thickens.

Remove the sauce from the heat and stir in the fontina, Gouda, and Cheddar until melted. Whisk in the sour cream. Add the pasta and stir until well coated. Return the saucepan to medium heat and add ½ cup of the reserved pasta water, stirring to combine. If the sauce is still too thick, add the rest of the water. Cook over medium heat for just a few minutes, until the pasta is al dente.

Transfer the mac and cheese to the prepared baking dish. In a small bowl, toss together the cracker crumbs, melted butter, and bacon and sprinkle the mixture on top of the mac and cheese. Broil for 3 to 4 minutes, until the topping is golden brown and the bacon is fragrant. Remove from the oven and serve right away.

Ginger-Glazed Carrots

Ginger is a wonderful mood booster. Its sweet heat is a wake-up call for the palate and the mind, and it has properties that settle the stomach, great for when stress is at its height. The carrot is a mild vegetable that has natural sugars, which are also mood improvers, but no refined sugars. As a side dish, these glazed carrots are the perfect pairing to almost any meal. They are easy to make, too, so the preparation won't add any unnecessary complications to your life.

1 pound carrots, peeled
3 tablespoons unsalted butter
1 teaspoon kosher salt, plus more to taste
1 teaspoon granulated sugar
1 tablespoon ginger jam (see Note on page 197)

1 teaspoon grated fresh ginger
¼ teaspoon freshly ground white pepper, plus more as needed (optional)
⅓ cup homemade or store-bought low-sodium chicken stock or vegetable stock

Cut the carrots into ¼-inch slices on the diagonal and transfer them to a medium high-sided skillet. In a small bowl, mix the butter, salt, sugar, ginger jam, fresh ginger, white pepper, if using, and stock until thoroughly combined. Add this ginger glaze to the skillet.

Bring the mixture to a boil over medium-high heat. Reduce the heat to medium-low and cook until the carrots are fork tender and the glaze has reduced enough to just coat the carrot. Taste and add salt and pepper as needed. Serve hot.

Twice-Baked Potatoes

SERVES 4 AS A SIDE

A good baked potato is a delicious thing, but a twice-baked potato is heart healing. While baked potatoes are delicious, the added techniques here give you a little more quiet time in the kitchen to settle the mind in prep work, and the finished product feels a bit more special. Packed with flavor, this dish is the perfect middle ground between mashed potatoes and baked potatoes.

5 large russet potatoes
2 tablespoons grapeseed or canola oil
Kosher salt and freshly ground black pepper,
   to taste

4 tablespoons unsalted butter
2 cups grated sharp Cheddar, divided
1 cup sour cream
2 tablespoons finely chopped chives

Preheat the oven to 400°F. Brush the outside of the potatoes with the oil, season with salt and pepper, and place on a baking sheet.

Bake for about 1 hour, or until the potatoes are fork tender. Leave the oven on, but remove the potatoes. With a fork, prick the tops of the potatoes a couple of times to release steam, and set them aside to cool slightly.

As soon as they are cool enough to handle, peel 1 potato and place its flesh into a large mixing bowl. With the remaining 4 potatoes, cut ¼ inch from the long side of each and remove the peel, adding the small bit of flesh to the potato in the bowl. Using a spoon, carefully remove the flesh from the middle of each potato, leaving a ¼-inch-thick shell all the way around and on the bottom. Add the scooped flesh to the bowl.

Add the butter to the bowl and mix with the potatoes until melted. Add 1 cup of the Cheddar and the sour cream and stir until the mixture looks like very chunky mashed potatoes. Taste and add salt and pepper as needed. Stir in the chives.

Divide the potato mixture into 4 equal portions. Use them to fill the 4 potato shells, making sure the filling nicely overflows on top of each shell. Divide the remaining 1 cup of Cheddar among the tops of each potato and press lightly to adhere.

Return the potatoes to the baking sheet and bake for 15 minutes, until the potatoes are heated through and the cheese is melted and golden. Serve right away.

NOTE: You can make these potatoes a day ahead, but skip the final baking and chill in the fridge instead. Before you want to serve, add the final dose of Cheddar on top and then reheat them in a 300°F oven for 20 to 30 minutes.

Salted-Caramel Banana Pudding

SERVES 12

Many people rave about the famous Magnolia Bakery in New York for its cupcakes, but the banana pudding is the dessert that haunts my dreams. The shop's version is at once lighter, fluffier, and richer than most versions. Often when we think of comfort foods, we are thinking of "nursery food," the foods of our early childhood that evoke memories and safety, security, and a sense of easy living and joy. Nothing does this better than a pudding, whether it's the fancy cooked puddings of your grandmother, the instant puddings you helped your mother make, or even the packaged pudding cups that always felt like a special treat in your lunchbox. This dish is an amped-up version, but the result is the same. You do need to make it the day before you want to eat it, but it is worth the planning ahead. Using the Magnolia Bakery technique as a jumping-off point, this version includes layers of salted caramel and a whipped cream topping to take it to the next level.

1 (14-ounce) can sweetened condensed milk
1½ cups ice-cold water
1 (3.4-ounce) package Jell-O Instant Vanilla
    Pudding mix
4½ cups heavy cream, divided
1 (12-ounce) box Nilla Wafers

4 small ripe bananas, sliced (4 cups)
1 cup caramel topping, such as Mrs.
    Richardson's
½ teaspoon flaky sea salt, such as Maldon,
    divided
Grated Nilla Wafers, for garnish (optional)

In a large bowl, thoroughly combine the sweetened condensed milk and water with a whisk until the sweetened condensed milk is completely dissolved. It should be about the consistency of whole milk. Add the pudding mix and continue to whisk for 2 to 3 more minutes, making sure that there are no lumps or pockets of unblended powder. Place a sheet of plastic wrap right on the top of the pudding, pressing it down so that there is no air; this will prevent the pudding from forming a skin. Store in the fridge for at least 4 hours or as long as overnight. When you put the pudding in the fridge, put the bowl of your stand mixer or whatever metal bowl you are going to use to whip the cream in as well, so that it is nice and chilled when you are ready for it!

When you are ready to begin assembly, remove the pudding mixture from the fridge. Let it rest at room temperature while you prepare your ingredients. In the pre-chilled bowl of your stand mixer fitted with the whisk attachment, whip 3 cups of the cream to stiff peaks. Be careful not to overwhip, or you will make butter! Set the whipped cream aside.

CONTINUED ▷

Salted-Caramel Banana Pudding
CONTINUED

Whisk the pudding mixture a bit to make it smooth and easier to work with, then add about one-third of the whipped cream to the pudding, whisking to combine the ingredients and lighten the pudding. Add the lightened pudding mixture to the bowl with the rest of the whipped cream. Fold the pudding mixture into the whipped cream with a rubber spatula until completely combined, being careful not to deflate it too much. Set it aside.

In a 3-quart bowl, deep casserole dish, or deep, disposable foil pan, layer one-third of the wafers followed by one-third of the banana slices. In a microwave, heat the caramel topping for 20 seconds, until it is just pourable. Drizzle half of the warm caramel over the bananas and wafers. Sprinkle with half of the salt. Add one-third of the pudding mixture and spread it over the top. Repeat this process once and then finish it off with the final layers of wafers, bananas, and pudding, in that order. Cover and store in the fridge for at least 8 hours or overnight.

Before serving, in the bowl of your stand mixer whip the remaining 1½ cups of cream to soft peaks. Remove the pudding from the fridge and top with the whipped cream. Garnish the whipped cream with the grated wafers, if using. I find a large spoon is the easiest way to serve.

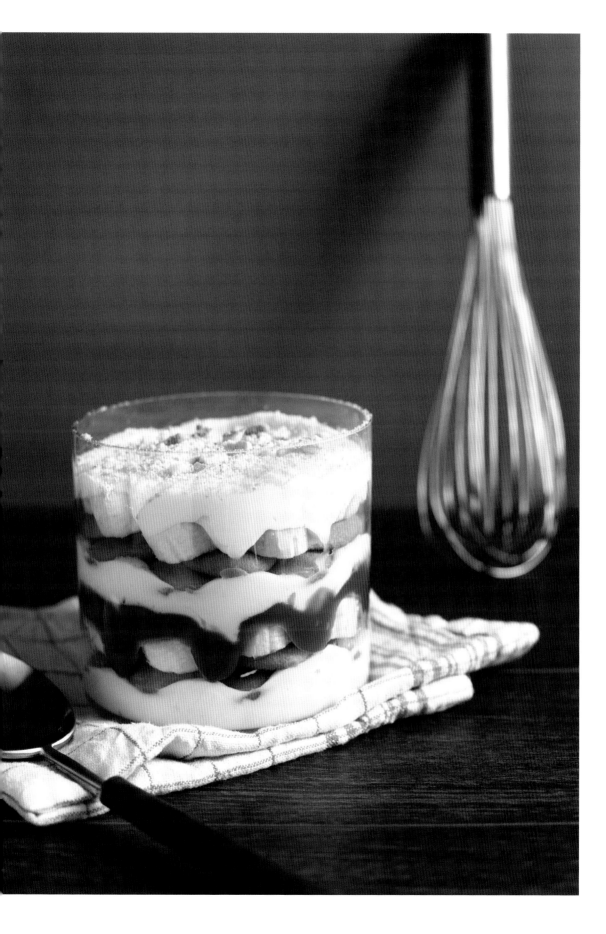

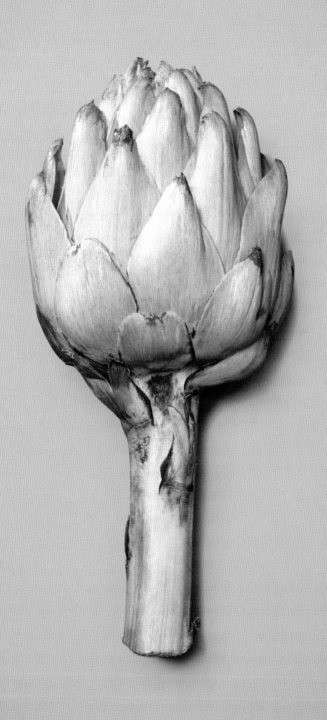

CHAPTER 4:
Environmental Wellness

ENVIRONMENTAL WELLNESS IS ABOUT **PRESERVING**.
It is about protecting the natural resources that we all need to sustain life and
healthy living. The World Health Organization estimates that, by the year
2050, the global population will increase by 25 percent. At the same time, the
earth's natural resources will not. Further, the United States accounts for only
5 percent of the world's population yet consumes 25 percent of the world's natural resources. We can and must do better! Environmental wellness incorpo-
rates the popular "three Rs": reduce, reuse, and recycle. I include two more Rs:
renew (replacing what we use, like planting a vegetable after harvesting one)
and repurpose (using resources for other needs, such as turning a plastic bottle
into a planter). While some consider this dimension to be more about community and less about oneself, I disagree. By doing your part to preserve the
earth's resources, you are taking care of both others and yourself. Think about
how good it feels to complete a long-overdue home project—like cleaning out
the kitchen cupboards. You feel refreshed, even renewed! This is how it feels to
nurture your environmental well-being.

COOKING for your environmental well-being takes many
forms. In this chapter, I've included primary recipes that make
large amounts of food. Each one is followed by a secondary
recipe that makes use of the leftovers. This gives you a concrete
way to avoid wasting food by repurposing your meals before
they spoil. When shopping for ingredients, select those that include pasture-raised meats and Certified Organic veggies, both
of which lessen our food system's impact on the environment.
Wherever possible in these recipes, I recommend products that
are organic, pasture raised, or grass fed. If you have access to
farmers' markets where you can buy straight from the producers,
so much the better! When preparing your food, do your best to
reuse kitchen items, such as mixing bowls and utensils, creating
less to wash and less water to waste. Think ahead when warming
the oven to try and reuse it for other parts of your prep before it
cools down. Cooking for your environmental well-being means
being mindful of what you use, how you use it, and how you can
be as efficient as possible.

EATING for your environmental well-being means doing so in a manner that reduces your environmental footprint. *Reducing* the amount of food you consume is not only good for the environment, but it also contributes to other factors of wellness by saving you money (financial) and maintaining your desired weight (physical). *Reusing* food by eating leftovers helps ensure that waste is kept to a minimum. *Recycling* everything that you cannot reuse or repurpose is an essential part of the process. For example, food packaging that is safe only for one-time use should be recycled. Look for the small triangular symbol on the bottom of cans, bottles, and other packaging. There will be a number inside of the triangle that represents how easy it is to recycle—the lower the number, the better. Regardless, if you cannot reuse or repurpose it, recycle it! *Renewing* what you eat means turning leftover dishes into completely new taste sensations by incorporating them into a new dish. Nothing tastes better than using your own homegrown ingredients in your meals. *Repurpose* what you don't eat by composting, feeding the birds, or making pet food from those leftovers that are not yet spoiled and/or moldy, but no longer suited for human consumption. I know you will enjoy the environmental benefits from the following delicious recipes.

Cooking for your environmental well-being means being mindful of what you use, how you use it, and how you can be as efficient as possible.

White Bean Dip

Entertaining can be great, but it can also be wasteful. A lot of the items we serve for guests at parties get dumped at the end of the event because there isn't something else to do with them. Not so with a veggie and dip platter, as long as the dip is this one! The leftovers can be made into a delicious soup. And even if the veggies are a bit wilted, you can always purée them in your blender for your own take on V8 vegetable juice!

½ cup + 2 tablespoons extra virgin olive oil, divided
1 large onion, sliced
2 (15-ounce) cans cannellini beans or other white beans, drained
Freshly squeezed juice of 1½ lemons
1 clove garlic

1 tablespoon fresh thyme leaves
Kosher salt and freshly ground black pepper, to taste
2–3 cups sliced raw vegetables, such as carrots, celery, jicama, cucumber, red bell peppers, and mushrooms

In a medium skillet set over medium-low heat, heat 2 tablespoons of the oil until it shimmers. Add the onions and cook, stirring occasionally, for 15 to 20 minutes, until they are deep brown. Remove the skillet from the heat and transfer the caramelized onions to a plate lined with paper towels to drain and cool.

Transfer the caramelized onions to the bowl of a food processor. Add the remaining ½ cup of oil and the beans, lemon juice, garlic, and thyme. Taste and add salt and pepper as needed. Blend until smooth and creamy.

Transfer 1 cup of the dip to an airtight container and save in the fridge for a future use. Serve the remaining dip with the raw vegetables.

WHITE BEAN CHOWDER

SERVES 4 TO 6

4 cups homemade or store-bought
   low-sodium chicken stock,
   divided
4 tablespoons unsalted butter
1 pound yellow onions, diced
1 head fennel, diced
1 teaspoon kosher salt, plus more
   to taste
¼ cup all-purpose flour
2 cups half and half or 2% milk (do
   not go leaner)

1 pound Yukon gold potatoes,
   peeled and diced
2 (15-ounce) cans white beans,
   drained and rinsed
2–3 sprigs fresh thyme
1 cup leftover White Bean Dip
   (page 90)
Freshly ground black pepper, to
   taste
Extra virgin olive oil, for garnish
Chopped fresh thyme, for garnish
   (optional)

In a small saucepan set over medium-high heat, heat 1 cup of the
chicken stock to a simmer, then reduce the heat to low. In a small
stockpot set over medium-high heat, heat the butter until it stops
foaming. Add the onions, fennel, and salt. Sauté for 2 minutes
until the onions are translucent and just the slightest bit browned,
but not deeply caramelized.

Sprinkle in the flour and stir until the flour and butter are well
blended. Cook, stirring constantly, for 2 minutes, until the flour
starts to smell nutty. Whisk in the simmering stock, until the mixture is fully incorporated and begins to thicken like a sauce. Whisk
in the remaining 3 cups of stock and the half and half. Add the
potatoes, beans, and thyme and bring to a gentle simmer.

Reduce the heat to medium-low, stir in the dip, and simmer for
10 minutes. Reduce the heat to low and continue to simmer for
another 30 minutes. Taste and add salt and pepper as needed.

Portion into bowls. Garnish with the oil and thyme, if using. Serve
immediately.

> **NOTE:** To store leftover soup, let it cool and transfer it to an airtight
> container. Refrigerate for up to 3 days or freeze for up to 2 months.
> Gently reheat it before serving.

Roasted Tomato Soup

In the summer, if you don't have a glut of tomatoes in your own garden, I bet you have a friend who does! And while we love those perfect, gorgeous tomatoes in salads, there is always a ton of crop that is sun split, slightly bruised, or just less than pretty. But that doesn't mean those tomatoes aren't just as delicious. You can't find a better way to eliminate garden waste than to use the more homely or imperfect veggies in a soup. This soup is wonderful hot or cold, freezes beautifully, and can be converted into several other recipes, so you can use up those fresh tomatoes at their peak.

8 pounds ripe tomatoes (a combination of plum and beefsteak is best)
¼ cup extra virgin olive oil
1 medium Vidalia onion, or 4 large shallots, diced
2 tablespoons herbes de Provence

1 tablespoon kosher salt, plus more to taste
1 teaspoon freshly ground black pepper, plus more to taste
Crème fraîche, for garnish
Chopped fresh mint, for garnish

Preheat the oven to 250°F. Grease 2 half-sheet pans and set aside.

Halve the tomatoes and place in a bowl. Add the oil and toss to coat. Transfer the tomatoes, cut-side down, to the prepared pans. Add the onion on top of the tomatoes. Season with the herbes de Provence, salt, and pepper. Roast for 1½ to 2 hours, until the tomato skins are loose and the flesh is soft. Remove from the oven.

Peel off the tomato skins and discard. Transfer everything from the pans, including all the juices, to a large bowl. Using an immersion blender, or pulsing in batches in a blender, blend the mixture into chunky soup. Taste and add salt and pepper as needed.

Transfer 3 cups of the soup to an airtight container and save in the fridge for a future use. Serve the remaining soup hot, garnished with crème fraîche and mint. If serving the soup cold, chill it in the fridge for 2 hours before garnishing.

PASTA WITH HOMEMADE TOMATO SAUCE

SERVES 6

1 tablespoon extra virgin olive oil
1 clove garlic, minced
1 shallot, minced
3 cups leftover Roasted Tomato
   Soup (page 92)

½ cup fresh basil leaves, chopped
1 pound pasta of your choice,
   cooked according to package
   directions

In a medium saucepan set over medium-high heat, heat the oil until it shimmers. Add the garlic and shallot and sauté until they are translucent but not browned. Add the Roasted Tomato Soup and cook until heated through. Stir in the basil. Serve over the pasta.

Greek Salad

A Greek salad can easily become an entrée with the addition of a can of good tuna, sliced grilled chicken breast, or a pair of perfectly cooked lamb chops. But a dressed salad usually doesn't last a second day. However, I've figured out how to turn these leftovers into a pasta salad to extend its life—a great trick!

¼ medium red onion, chopped
3 tablespoons extra virgin olive oil
1½ tablespoons freshly squeezed lemon juice
1 clove garlic, minced
½ teaspoon dried oregano
¼ teaspoon fine sea salt

¼ teaspoon freshly ground black pepper
3 tomatoes, cut into 1-inch cubes
½ cucumber, seeded and cut into 1-inch chunks
4 ounces feta, diced medium
16 Kalamata olives, pitted and halved

Soak the onion in a small bowl of cold, salted water for 10 minutes; this takes the harsh bite out if it. Drain the onion and pat it dry with paper towels. Set aside.

To make the dressing, in a small bowl place the oil, lemon juice, garlic, oregano, salt, and pepper and give everything a good whisk. You are not looking for an emulsification here; it is more of a broken vinaigrette.

In a large bowl, combine the onion, tomatoes, cucumber, feta, and olives. Add the dressing and toss.

Transfer 2 cups of the salad to an airtight container and save in the fridge for a future use. Serve the remaining salad right away.

GREEK PASTA SALAD

SERVES 4 AS A SIDE

¼ cup extra virgin olive oil

2 tablespoons freshly squeezed lemon juice

½ teaspoon kosher salt, plus more to taste

8 ounces dried penne, rotini, or orecchiette, cooked in well-salted water according to package directions and drained

2 cups leftover Greek Salad (page 94), with juices

1 tablespoon chopped fresh dill

2 tablespoons chopped fresh flat-leaf parsley

Freshly ground black pepper, to taste

2 tablespoons toasted pine nuts, for garnish (see Note on page 159)

In a large bowl, mix together the oil, lemon juice, and salt. Add the pasta and toss to combine. Let stand, tossing occasionally, at room temperature for 30 minutes.

Add the Greek Salad and combine well. Let stand, tossing occasionally, for another 20 minutes, so that the pasta soaks up the dressing and juices from the Greek Salad. Add the dill and parsley. Taste and add salt and pepper as needed.

Garnish with the pine nuts and serve right away.

> **NOTE:** If not serving right away, transfer the salad to the fridge. However, it's best if you take it out and let it rest at room temperature for 30 to 45 minutes before serving. You can substitute 1 pound of cooked, cubed potatoes for the cooked pasta for a different take on a potato salad!

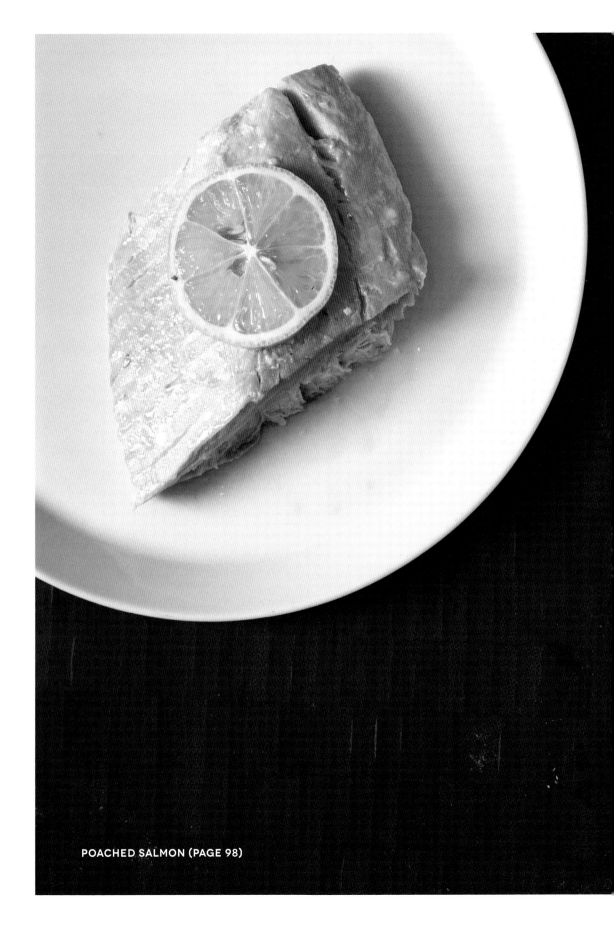

POACHED SALMON (PAGE 98)

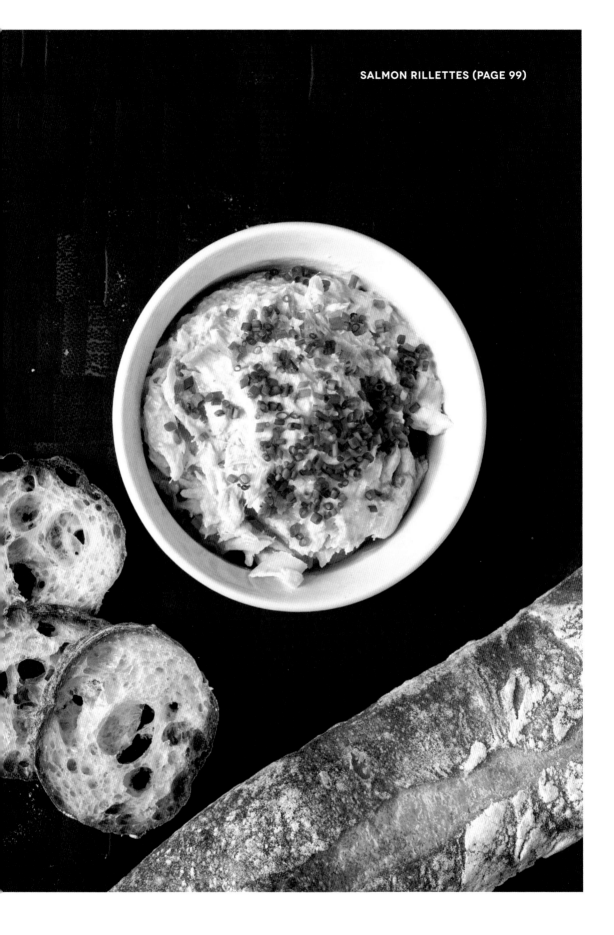
SALMON RILLETTES (PAGE 99)

Poached Salmon

We all know that leftover fish is a complicated thing; since it doesn't last very long or reheat well, it can be hard to find a good way to use it the next day. This duo of salmon dishes offers a creative solution. The first is adapted from the best: Eric Ripert, arguably the world's top seafood chef. His poaching technique results in a texture that is sublime on its own and also ideal for the luxurious second recipe, a version of salmon rillettes inspired by the award-winning Thomas Keller. Rillettes are a traditional French technique for preserving meat. While this version uses dairy instead of the customary animal fat to bind the fish, it is no less rich and delicious than its meatier counterparts. And it can take your leftover fish and make it into something that can last for five or six days! I have made both of these sophisticated dishes a bit simpler for the home cook, but they lose nothing in flavor.

3 cups room temperature + ¼ cup cold water, divided
4½ tablespoons all-purpose flour
1 teaspoon sea salt, plus more to taste
½ teaspoon freshly ground black pepper, plus more to taste

½ cup dry white wine
Zest of 1 orange
Zest of 1 lemon
4 (8-ounce) wild-caught salmon fillets, skinned and pin bones removed (your fishmonger can do this for you)

In a large skillet set over medium-high heat, bring the 3 cups of room-temperature water to a boil. Meanwhile, in a small bowl whisk the flour into the ¼ cup of cold water until fully blended with no lumps. Add the salt and pepper.

When the water in the skillet is boiling, quickly whisk in the flour mixture. This thickens the water slightly—which is different from most poaching recipes—creating a more supportive, gentle environment for the fish. When the mixture is about the texture of heavy cream, stir in the white wine, orange zest, and lemon zest. Continue to boil until the liquid has thickened to the texture of gravy, and then reduce the heat to low.

Season both sides of the fish with salt and pepper, and gently slide the fillets into the poaching liquid. Cook for 4 to 5 minutes; the fish should feel slightly firm to the touch but still a bit soft in the middle.

Remove the skillet from the heat to a cold burner and let the fish rest in the poaching liquid for 1 to 2 minutes.

Using a spatula, transfer 2 of the fillets to an airtight container and save in the fridge for a future use. Gently transfer the remaining fillets to a serving platter and serve.

> **NOTE**: This dish is great with rice and steamed asparagus, or over a salad dressed with a Dijon mustard vinaigrette.

SALMON RILLETTES

1 stick unsalted butter, room temperature, divided
1 shallot, minced
1 tablespoon cream cheese, room temperature
1 tablespoon freshly squeezed lemon juice
1½ teaspoons extra virgin olive oil
1 egg yolk, lightly beaten

2 leftover Poached Salmon fillets (page 98), flaked into large pieces
Kosher salt and freshly ground black pepper, to taste
2 tablespoons minced chives, for garnish
Crackers or toasted baguette slices, for serving

In a medium pan set over low heat, melt 1 tablespoon of the butter until the foaming subsides. Add the shallot and cook, stirring, until it is translucent and soft but not browned. Remove from the heat and set aside to cool.

In a medium bowl, combine the remaining 7 tablespoons of butter and the cream cheese. Blend with a spatula until completely mixed. Stir in the cooled shallots. Add the lemon juice and oil, stirring well to combine. Add the egg yolk and stir until you have a cohesive mixture.

Place the Poached Salmon in a large bowl. Gently fold the butter-shallot mixture into the fish until all of the salmon pieces are coated. Don't overmix, or you will get a smooth paste instead of a chunky spread. Taste and add salt and pepper as needed.

Transfer the salmon rillettes to a serving bowl and place a piece of plastic wrap directly onto the surface. Transfer to the fridge and chill for at least 3 hours or as long as overnight.

Garnish with the chives and serve cold with the crackers.

> **NOTE**: If you want the rillettes to last longer in the fridge, smooth them into an airtight container and top with ¼ inch of clarified butter. When the butter hardens in the fridge, it will help keep the rillettes fresh for a few extra days.

Asian Caramel Chicken Thighs

When compared to chicken breast, boneless, skinless chicken thighs have only 2 calories more per ounce. Since most people ask for boneless, skinless breasts, thigh meat is both plentiful and less expensive. Every dish you cook with thighs balances out another person who only uses breast meat. But whether you are using breast meat or thigh meat, it is easy to get into a chicken rut. I recently came across a version of this recipe in *Cook's Illustrated* magazine. I was very intrigued, since I was a sucker for sweet-and-sour chicken when I was a kid. This seemed like a fun way to try a new chicken dish with a bit of sweetness and geared toward a more grown-up palate. I like to serve these chicken thighs with steamed rice on the side or over stir-fried greens. The second-night dinner is a terrific way to use up the leftovers and introduce a whole new taste sensation.

⅔ cup water, divided
⅓ cup firmly packed dark brown sugar
3 tablespoons fish sauce
1½ tablespoons grated fresh ginger
Zest of 1 orange

2 tablespoons freshly squeezed orange juice
¼–½ teaspoon red pepper flakes
2 pounds boneless, skinless chicken thighs, cut into bite-sized pieces

In a medium saucepan set over medium-high heat, bring ⅓ cup of the water to a boil. Add the brown sugar and cook, stirring constantly, until the sugar is melted and the mixture has become a thick caramel, 6 to 8 minutes.

Reduce the heat to medium-low. Stir in the fish sauce, ginger, orange zest, orange juice, and red pepper flakes. Slowly drizzle in the remaining ⅓ cup of water, stirring constantly, until the mixture comes to a gentle simmer. You should end up with a thick sauce, about the consistency of light cream.

Add the chicken and gently stir until all of the chicken is coated in the sauce. Cook, stirring frequently, for 12 to 15 minutes, until the chicken is cooked through. Be sure to watch the heat so that the mixture doesn't boil but remains at a simmer.

Transfer half (1 pound) of the caramel chicken to an airtight container and store in the fridge for a future use. Remove the remaining caramel chicken from the heat, transfer to a platter, and serve.

ASIAN CHICKEN WRAPS

SERVES 4

4 tablespoons canola oil, divided
½ cup minced yellow onion
½ cup bamboo shoots, julienned
1 teaspoon grated fresh ginger
1 pound leftover Asian Caramel
   Chicken Thighs (page 100)
1 jalapeño, minced
1 tablespoon fish sauce
2 teaspoons dark brown sugar
2 teaspoons soy sauce

¼ teaspoon freshly ground black
   pepper
1 cup fresh cilantro leaves
1 tablespoon freshly squeezed lime
   juice
¼ cup chopped roasted peanuts
Iceberg, romaine, or butter lettuce
   leaf cups, for serving
1 lime, quartered, for serving

In a large nonstick skillet set over medium-high heat, heat 2 tablespoons of the oil until it shimmers. Add the onion and sauté for 2 minutes. Add the bamboo shoots and continue to cook for 1 minute. Add the ginger and mix well, cooking for 30 seconds. Transfer the mixture to a small bowl and set aside.

In the same pan, still over medium-high heat, add the remaining 2 tablespoons of oil and the Asian Caramel Chicken Thighs. Cook, stirring constantly, for 2 minutes, just until the chicken is heated through. Add the jalapeño and cook 1 minute. Add the bamboo shoot mixture, fish sauce, sugar, soy sauce, and black pepper and stir. Cook for 3 to 4 minutes, until thoroughly heated. Remove from the heat.

Stir in the cilantro leaves and lime juice, mixing well. Garnish with the chopped peanuts. To assemble, put about 2 tablespoons of the chicken mixture into each lettuce cup and roll them up. Serve with the lime wedges.

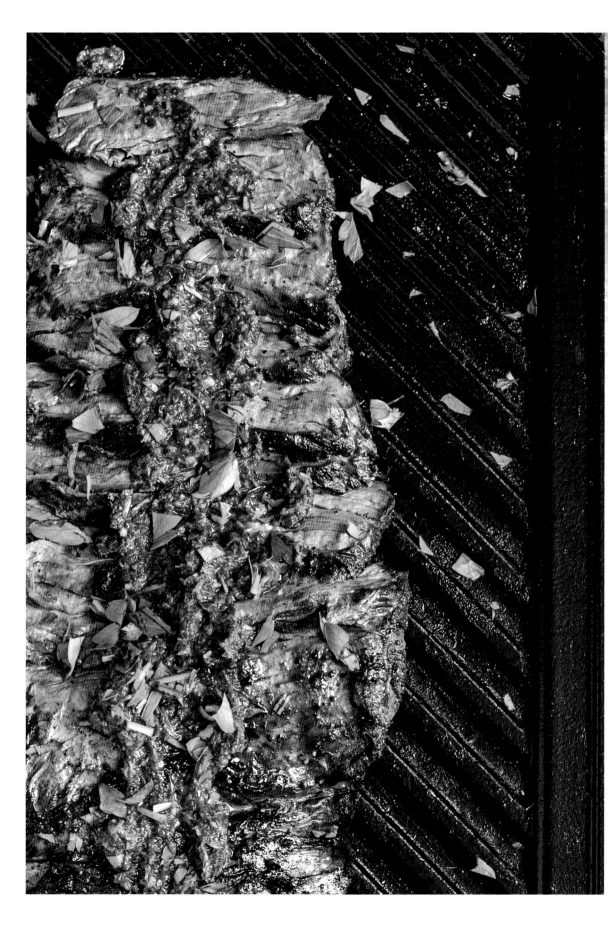

Skirt Steaks with Shallot Chimichurri

SERVES 4 (WITH 2 LEFTOVER STEAKS)

Skirt steaks are one of the best lean and affordable cuts of beef to add to your repertoire. They also stand up to a second-day reheat beautifully. If you buy organic, grass-fed beef, you can feel good about incorporating red meat in your diet, especially when you know you will get two meals out of it. Organic, grass-fed beef creates a much smaller carbon footprint. While the original recipe that I found in the *New York Times* used a shallot butter garnish, skirt steaks are a great meat to pair with a less fatty and more deeply flavored chimichurri. This version of chimichurri uses those shallots instead of garlic, an interesting twist on the typical preparation.

6 (6-ounce) lean skirt steaks, preferably
    organic and grass fed
Kosher salt and freshly ground black pepper,
    to taste

1 recipe Shallot Chimichurri (recipe follows),
    for serving

Season the steaks on both sides with salt and pepper. Heat a large nonstick skillet or grill pan over high heat. Spray both sides of the steaks with nonstick spray.

Cook the steaks for 3 to 4 minutes on the first side, until thoroughly browned. Turn the steaks and cook on the other side until lightly browned, 2 to 3 minutes, until an instant-read thermometer inserted into the thickest part of the meat registers 130°F for medium rare. Transfer the steaks to a plate and let them rest for 10 minutes.

Transfer 2 of the steaks to an airtight container and save in the fridge for a future use. Serve the remaining 4 steaks hot with a spoonful of the Shallot Chimichurri. You should have some chimichurri left over.

Shallot Chimichurri

4½ tablespoons finely chopped shallots
1½ teaspoons fresh thyme leaves
1½ tablespoons red wine vinegar

6 tablespoons finely chopped fresh flat-leaf
    parsley
6 tablespoons extra virgin olive oil

Place all the ingredients into a blender. Pulse until the mixture is a chunky salsa. Store in an airtight container in the fridge until ready to use, up to 5 days.

SECOND-DAY FAJITAS

SERVES 4

1 tablespoon olive oil
1 medium yellow onion, sliced
1 poblano pepper, seeded and thinly sliced
2 leftover Skirt Steaks (page 103), sliced into ½-inch strips across the grain
2 tablespoons leftover Shallot Chimichurri (page 103)

2 tablespoons chopped fresh cilantro
8 steamed wheat tortillas, for serving
Shredded Chihuahua cheese or crumbled queso fresco, for serving
Sour cream, for serving
Sliced avocado, for serving (optional)

In a small skillet set over medium-high heat, heat the oil until it shimmers. Add the onion and pepper and sauté until they begin to develop a good char. Transfer to a bowl and set aside. Keep the heat on.

In a large bowl, toss the steak strips with the Shallot Chimichurri and cilantro. Add everything to the hot skillet and cook for 2 to 3 minutes, until the mixture is heated through and the steak slices brown a bit. Transfer to a bowl.

To serve, place some slices of steak and some of the onions and peppers into each of the tortillas. Garnish with the cheese, sour cream, and avocado, if using, and serve.

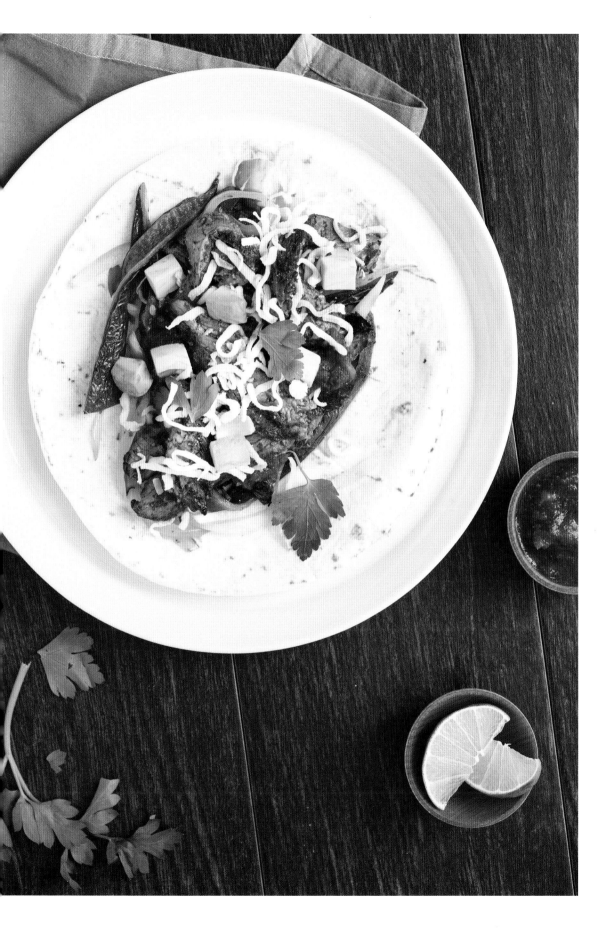

Pork Chops Oreganata

Pork chops are a quick and easy dinner option, but the act of reheating them usually renders them tough and dry, which often means that leftovers just get discarded. The first recipe is inspired by one from Food.com. However, I added a crucial step: dry-brining. It's necessary if you are going to use pork leftovers in a stew and want them to stand up to being twice-cooked. Dry-brining helps the chops retain moisture, which makes them more succulent in the first recipe and keeps them tender for the second! By turning these leftovers into a rich stew, you get a second meal out of your chops, without getting pork jerky! And the stew freezes beautifully if you don't want pork two nights in a row.

10 (4–5-ounce) boneless pork loin chops
1 tablespoon kosher salt
Freshly ground black pepper, to taste
3 tablespoons extra virgin olive oil
½ cup dry white wine

5 cloves garlic, minced
3 tablespoons minced yellow onion
½ cup + 2 tablespoons fresh oregano leaves, chopped
½ teaspoon dried thyme

Season both sides of the chops with the salt and pepper and set aside in a large covered baking dish for 1 hour at room temperature to dry-brine. It is fine to stack them in two layers. This will get great flavor into the chops and help them retain moisture.

In a large nonstick skillet set over medium-high heat, heat the oil until it shimmers. In two batches, cook the pork chops for 3 to 4 minutes per side, until golden brown, and transfer them to a clean baking dish. (Do not put them back in the baking dish they were in for the dry brine! Always keep raw and cooked foods separate for food safety.)

Reduce the heat to medium and add the wine. Bring to a boil and let it reduce for 1 minute. Add the garlic and onion and cook until the onion is translucent and the mixture is slightly thickened. Stir in the oregano and thyme and cook for 1 more minute.

Pour the sauce over the pork chops. Transfer 4 of the chops to an airtight container and save in the fridge for a future use.

Serve the remaining 6 chops hot with any extra sauce spooned over.

> **NOTE:** This stew lends itself to garnishes, and it is fun for people to be able to personalize their bowls. Think about setting out a garnish station with tortilla strips, cabbage, lime wedges, sour cream, avocado cubes, diced radishes, cilantro leaves, and minced sweet onion for a real party!

MEXICAN PORK STEW

SERVES 4

4 leftover Pork Chops Oreganata
  (page 106)
½ yellow onion, diced
4 cloves garlic, minced
2 dried bay leaves
Zest and freshly squeezed juice of
  1 orange
1 (12-ounce) bottle beer (whatever
  you have on hand)
5 tablespoons chili powder (ancho
  if you can find it)
½ yellow onion, chopped
1 carrot, peeled and diced
2 ribs celery, diced

3 whole cloves garlic
Kosher salt and freshly ground
  black pepper, to taste
Pinch red pepper flakes, or 1–2
  dashes hot sauce (optional)
1 (19-ounce) can hominy, drained
  and rinsed
1 (15-ounce) can light red kidney
  beans, drained and rinsed
2 tablespoons fresh oregano leaves
1 teaspoon red wine vinegar
Shredded cabbage and fried tortilla
  strips, for garnish

In a large stockpot, combine the pork chops, diced onion, minced garlic, bay leaves, and orange zest and juice. Add water to cover everything by 1 inch and set the pot over medium-high heat. Bring to a simmer and cook for about 30 minutes, until the pork is very tender and can be easily shredded with a fork. If the pork isn't ready, continue to simmer for an additional 10 to 15 minutes.

Transfer the pork to a cutting board. Using two forks, pull the pork into bite-sized pieces. Set aside. Strain the stock and discard the solids, return the strained stock to the pot, and place it over medium-high heat. Add the beer and bring the mixture to a boil. Reduce the heat to medium-low and add the chili powder, chopped onion, carrot, celery, and whole garlic cloves.

Simmer for 10 minutes to let the flavors meld, then taste and add salt and pepper as needed. If it isn't as spicy as you'd like, add the red pepper flakes. Add the reserved pork, hominy, and beans, stirring well to combine. Bring the stew back to a simmer and continue cooking for an additional 30 minutes. Stir in the oregano and vinegar and cook for 2 minutes, then taste one last time for seasoning and add salt and pepper as needed.

To serve, spoon the stew into bowls and garnish to your taste with shredded cabbage and fried tortilla strips.

Ponzu Tofu Steaks

This marinade is a great one to have in your back pocket; it works equally well for chicken or fish. Ponzu is a traditional Japanese sauce that is citrus based, with rice vinegar and seasonings. While traditionally it uses bonito flakes, or dried tuna flakes, as part of making the sauce, since this is a vegetarian recipe we have left them out. One way to embrace environmental wellness is to incorporate more vegetable cookery into your life, as it takes fewer resources to grow vegetables than it does to raise animals. Many people who don't want to embrace a vegetarian lifestyle full time can still participate in things like Meatless Mondays or commit to eating more meatless meals in order to reduce their carbon footprint. That's why, while this ponzu sauce works great with chicken or fish, I've suggested tofu here. Try switching up your dinner options once or twice a week and see if you don't feel better knowing you are doing a good thing for both yourself and the planet.

4 tablespoons freshly squeezed lime juice

4 tablespoons water

2 tablespoons grated fresh ginger

2 teaspoons sesame oil

4 tablespoons tamari or soy sauce

1 tablespoon rice vinegar

4 teaspoons granulated sugar

1 pound firm tofu, cut lengthwise into 8 equal slices

To make the ponzu sauce, in a small bowl combine all the ingredients except for the tofu and stir well.

Place the tofu slices, in a single layer, in a large baking dish. Add half of the ponzu sauce and let the tofu marinate for at least 1 hour at room temperature. Transfer the remaining ponzu sauce to an airtight container and save in the fridge for a future use.

Preheat the oven to 400°F.

Place the baking dish with the tofu slices in their marinade into the oven. Bake for 5 minutes, flip the tofu slices, and continue baking for 5 more minutes.

Remove the dish from the oven. Transfer 2 of the tofu slices to an airtight container and save in the fridge for a future use. Divide the remaining 6 slices between 6 plates and serve right away.

FRIED CAULIFLOWER RICE

SERVES 4

2½ tablespoons peanut oil, divided
2 leftover slices Ponzu Tofu Steaks
(page 108), cubed
½ teaspoon grated fresh ginger
1 teaspoon finely minced garlic
4 cups riced raw cauliflower (see
Note)
¼ cup minced yellow onion

¼ cup grated carrot
¼ cup frozen peas, thawed
¼ cup shredded cabbage
2 eggs, beaten (optional)
¼ cup leftover ponzu marinade
(page 108)
Soy sauce and freshly ground black
pepper, to taste

In a wok or a large sauté pan set over medium-high heat, heat 1 tablespoon of oil until it shimmers. Add the tofu cubes, toss them in the oil, and cook until browned. Transfer the tofu to a bowl and set aside. Add another 1 tablespoon of oil to the wok and reduce the heat to medium. When the oil shimmers, add the ginger and garlic and stir-fry for 20 seconds, just until they become fragrant.

Add the cauliflower, onion, carrot, peas, and cabbage. Increase the heat to high and stir-fry, moving the vegetables around constantly, until they are cooked but still have a little crunch, about 3 minutes. Transfer the cooked vegetables to the bowl with the tofu.

Add the remaining ½ tablespoon of oil to the wok, and stir in the eggs, if using, scrambling them into large curds. Add the vegetables and tofu back to the pan, along with the ponzu marinade, and continue to stir-fry until everything is combined and hot. Taste and add soy sauce and pepper as needed.

Transfer to a large serving bowl and serve hot.

NOTE: You can often find riced cauliflower in the produce section of your grocery store. If you can't buy it prepped, you can pulse cauliflower florets in your food processor to get the texture of rice.

Polenta with Vegetables and Cheese

SERVES 4 (WITH HALF LEFT OVER)

Back in the late 1980s, local Chicago restaurateur Ina Pinkney served a breakfast dish she called "vegetarian scrapple," which included a fried slice of polenta studded with corn and black beans and laced with Cheddar. Historically, scrapple was a dish made with leftover meat scraps mixed with cornmeal and chilled in a loaf pan. It was one of the original environmentally thoughtful dishes, using up scraps that would otherwise have gone to waste. These dishes use the same principle, but without meat. For added protein, serve with poached eggs and a green salad. This large batch of polenta allows you to put half of it into a loaf pan and store in the fridge for a second-day use as a breakfast, brunch, or lunch dish. You can use up any vegetables you like in these dishes, so feel free to dig around in your crisper drawer for things that are about to go bad and toss them in here.

2 quarts water
2 sticks unsalted butter
5 teaspoons kosher salt, plus more to taste
4 teaspoons freshly ground black pepper, plus more to taste
4 cups cornmeal

4 cups grated Cotija cheese
1 cup diced red bell pepper
1 cup diced zucchini
1 (15-ounce) can corn kernels, drained
2 (15-ounce) cans black beans, drained and rinsed

In a large pot set over medium-high heat, bring the water, butter, salt, and pepper to a boil. Reduce the heat to medium and whisk in the cornmeal in a steady stream until fully incorporated. Reduce the heat to medium-low and cook, stirring constantly, until the mixture has thickened and the cornmeal has lost its raw taste, about 10 minutes. Quickly whisk in the cheese until fully combined. Taste and add salt and pepper as needed.

Remove the pot from the heat. Add the bell pepper, zucchini, corn, and beans, folding them in with a spatula or wooden spoon.

Line a 9 × 5-inch loaf pan with plastic wrap. Pack in half of the hot polenta. You want to do this right away because the polenta will continue to thicken and stiffen as it cools, and you want to be able to make a nice loaf of the polenta for the next day. Smooth the top and cover tightly with plastic wrap, laying the plastic right on top of the polenta so that it touches the surface to prevent the top from drying out. Store in the fridge at least overnight, up to 2 days.

Serve the remaining polenta hot.

VEGETARIAN POLENTA CAKES

SERVES UP TO 8

1 loaf leftover Polenta with
  Vegetables and Cheese
  (page 110)
2 tablespoons ghee or grapeseed oil

8 tablespoons salsa, or as needed,
  for garnish (1 tablespoon per
  person)
16 eggs, or as needed, scrambled
  (2 per person)

Unmold the polenta loaf and remove the plastic wrap. Slice the loaf into about ¾-inch-thick slices (so you have about 8 slices, 1 slice per serving).

Heat a nonstick pan over medium-high heat, and add the ghee or grapeseed oil. Add the polenta slices and cook until they are golden brown and crispy on both sides.

Serve with salsa and scrambled eggs.

Mediterranean Vegetable Stew

Ratatouille is a classic southern French dish of stewed vegetables that is a wonderful side for almost any meat or fish. But, often the combination of vegetables is limited, and the dish can easily turn to mush. This stew takes the classic flavors of ratatouille and amps them up with some chickpeas for protein and the salty punch of capers. If you or your friends have gardens, it is usually tomatoes and zucchini that everyone always has too much of, and this is a terrific way to use them up! This is yet another recipe that turns a challenge (say, surplus veggies) into a cooking opportunity. Leftovers are delicious on their own, but adding a little spice and cooking eggs in them makes for an elegant brunch dish that will wow your family or guests.

½ cup extra virgin olive oil, plus more for garnish
1 large onion, diced
1 red bell pepper, seeded and diced
4 cloves garlic, minced
½ teaspoon red pepper flakes
2 tablespoons tomato paste
6 plum tomatoes, seeded and diced
1 zucchini, diced
1 yellow summer squash, diced

1 medium eggplant, diced
1 teaspoon kosher salt, plus more to taste
1 (15-ounce) can chickpeas, drained and rinsed
1 (15-ounce) can quartered baby artichokes, drained
1 tablespoon nonpareil capers
Freshly ground black pepper, to taste
½ cup chopped fresh basil
¼ cup chopped fresh flat-leaf parsley

In a large sauté pan set over medium-high heat, heat the oil until it shimmers. Add the onion and cook for about 2 minutes until it is translucent and softened. Add the bell pepper and cook until it softens. Stir in the garlic and red pepper flakes and cook, stirring constantly, for 1 minute. Add in the tomato paste and stir until it coats the mixture and browns slightly. Add the tomatoes, zucchini, squash, and eggplant and stir to combine. Add the salt and stir.

Reduce the heat to medium-low, cover, and cook for 10 minutes. Uncover the pan and stir in the chickpeas, artichokes, and capers. Continue cooking, uncovered, for another 10 minutes, or until the vegetables are soft but still holding their shape and not becoming a mush. Taste and add salt and pepper as needed. Stir in the basil and parsley and remove from the heat.

Transfer half of the stew to an airtight container and save in the fridge for a future use. Portion the remaining half into 4 bowls and garnish with a drizzle of the oil. Serve hot or at room temperature.

EGGS IN PURGATORY

1 tablespoon unsalted butter
2 tablespoons red or white wine
  (use whatever you happen to
  have)
½ recipe leftover Mediterranean
  Vegetable Stew (page 112)

Kosher salt and freshly ground
  black pepper, to taste
8 large eggs
Grated Parmesan, for garnish
Chopped fresh flat-leaf parsley or
  basil, for garnish

Preheat the oven to 350°F. Grease a 9 ×12-inch glass baking dish and set it aside.

In a large sauté pan set over medium-high heat, melt the butter. Add in the wine and stir to combine. Add the stew and stir, cooking gently for 5 minutes, until hot and somewhat thickened and dry. Taste and add salt and pepper as needed.

Transfer the stew into the prepared baking dish and spread it evenly over the bottom. Make 8 shallow divots in the stew, making sure to leave a thin layer of stew at the bottom of the divots. (You can also do this in individual ramekins.)

Gently crack 1 egg into each of the divots. Transfer to the oven and cook for 5 minutes, or until the eggs are cooked on top but the yolks are still liquid.

Serve 2 eggs with their stew base per person, gently lifting them out one at a time with a wide spatula. Garnish with grated Parmesan and parsley.

Artichoke Pasta

SERVES 4 AS A SIDE (WITH HALF LEFT OVER)

Pasta is a wonderful dinner, but leftovers often suffer with reheating. While some people love cold spaghetti for breakfast, second-day pastas are rarely a treat. This artichoke pasta is one of my favorite side dishes, really great for a romantic dinner. The next-day frittata is a version of one I saw from Mark Bittman. I had never seen a frittata with pasta in it before, but I realized that it would be a great dish to learn to make since it doesn't just use up the leftovers, it celebrates them! It is one of the easiest meals there is, and once you know the technique, you can use it with pretty much any leftover pasta you have.

1 pound linguini or spaghetti
1 tablespoon extra virgin olive oil
2 shallots, finely minced
1 cup homemade or store-bought low-sodium chicken stock
4 tablespoons artichoke purée or tapenade (available at gourmet stores), divided
6 cooked fresh artichoke bottoms, diced large
¼ cup dry sherry

1 teaspoon kosher salt
½ teaspoon freshly ground black pepper
2 tablespoons unsalted butter
4 tablespoons toasted pine nuts, for garnish (see Note on page 159)
2 tablespoons chopped fresh flat-leaf parsley, for garnish
4 tablespoons grated Parmesan, for garnish

In a large pot, cook the pasta in salted water according to the package directions. While the pasta is cooking, heat the oil in a large skillet set over medium-high heat. Add the shallots and cook until they have softened, about 2 minutes. Add the chicken stock and cook until the mixture is reduced by half, about 6 more minutes.

Whisk in 2 tablespoons of the artichoke purée. Add the artichoke bottoms, sherry, salt, and pepper. Cook for 3 to 4 minutes, until the artichoke pieces have heated through. Add the butter, swirling the pan to incorporate the butter smoothly.

Drain the pasta, reserving ½ cup of the cooking water.

Add the pasta and reserved cooking water to the sauce, tossing a few times to coat and heat through. Transfer half of the artichoke pasta to an airtight container and save in the fridge for a future use.

Transfer the remaining half of the artichoke pasta to a large serving bowl. Garnish with the pine nuts, parsley, and Parmesan. Serve right away.

ARTICHOKE–PASTA FRITTATA

SERVES 6

10 large eggs
1 cup grated Parmesan, plus more
   for garnish
¼ cup chopped fresh flat-leaf
   parsley or basil (optional)

½ recipe leftover Artichoke Pasta
   (page 114)
2 tablespoons extra virgin olive oil,
   plus more for garnish

Preheat the oven to 400°F.

In a large bowl, beat the eggs well. Add in the Parmesan and parsley, if using, and mix so that everything is well distributed. Add the artichoke pasta, mixing well so that the noodles and eggs become one soupy mass.

In a large nonstick, ovenproof skillet set over medium-high heat, heat the oil until it shimmers.

Pour the egg mixture into the skillet and cook, stirring so that small curds of egg form throughout, until the mixture begins to thicken slightly. Stop stirring and let the mixture settle, using a rubber spatula to keep the edges together. Reduce the heat to medium-low and continue to cook until the bottom of the frittata begins to feel like it is set; when you gently swirl the pan, it should move as one unit.

Transfer the pan to the oven and cook for 12 to 15 minutes, until the frittata no longer jiggles in the center.

Remove the frittata from the oven and immediately invert it onto a cutting board. Let sit for 10 minutes before slicing into wedges. Serve hot or at room temperature, with a drizzle of olive oil and grated Parmesan.

> **NOTE:** If you happen to have leftover marinara sauce hanging around your fridge, it makes a great garnish for this frittata and can turn it into a nice luncheon dish. Just warm the sauce before pouring it over the frittata slices.

Saffron Risotto

Many people think risotto is a complicated dish to make, and I used to be one of them! Despite being half Italian, I had never cooked risotto despite how much I love it, because I assumed it would be beyond my abilities. Then I saw a version of this recipe on *The Italian Dish* and realized that I was confusing complex with active. Risotto has only four simple steps: sauté the onion and rice, deglaze the pan with wine, slowly add the broth, and finish it with butter and cheese. It can actually be a very meditative dish to cook, and once you master the technique, you can alter the flavorings almost infinitely. Leftover risotto can easily be turned into a fun appetizer that freezes easily. I often make a large batch of risotto just to be able to make the arancini.

1 large pinch saffron threads
¼ cup white wine
6 cups homemade or store-bought low-sodium chicken broth, or as needed
4 tablespoons unsalted butter, cold, divided

2 shallots, minced
1 cup Arborio rice
½ cup grated Parmesan, plus more for garnish
Kosher salt and freshly ground black pepper, to taste

In a small bowl, put the saffron into the wine and set aside. In a medium pot set over medium heat, bring the broth to a simmer and then reduce the heat to low.

Place a large high-sided skillet or a chef's pan over medium-high heat. Add 2 tablespoons of the butter and melt it, but do not let it brown. Add the shallots and sauté until they are translucent. Add the rice and stir until every grain is coated with the butter and the grains appear slightly translucent and a bit golden.

Add the wine-saffron mixture and stir until the wine is completely absorbed. Add about 2 large ladles of the warm broth to the rice and begin stirring the mixture with a wooden spoon in gentle circles, being sure to get into the corners. The stirring doesn't need to be vigorous, just continuous. Stir the risotto constantly, letting the broth slowly absorb into the rice. When you can just start to see the bottom of the pan as you drag the spoon through, add another ladle of the broth and continue to stir. Continue this process for about 20 minutes, and then taste the rice for doneness; it should be toothsome—soft but slightly firm. If it's too firm, crunchy in the middle, or sticking in your teeth, continue adding broth, half a ladle at a time, and taste again when it's absorbed. The process can take anywhere from 20 to 40 minutes, and you might use all of the broth or have leftovers. The rice will tell you: you are looking for al dente grains suspended in a creamy sauce.

Remove the skillet from the heat and keep stirring the rice as it absorbs the last bit of broth. Add the Parmesan and stir to combine. Then add in the remaining 2 tablespoons of butter and stir vigorously to combine. You have to do this last bit with some speed, as you want to emulsify the butter into the rice and enhance the creaminess. If you simply let the butter melt or don't stir firmly enough, it will make the risotto greasy instead of creamy. Taste and add salt and pepper as needed.

Transfer 2 cups of the risotto to an airtight container and save in the fridge for a future use. Dish the remaining risotto into serving bowls. Garnish with the grated Parmesan and serve hot.

NOTE: The first key to risotto is letting the rice tell you what you need. Every batch is different, so this is less a recipe than it is a technique. The amounts listed here are only guidelines. For example, if you don't have shallots, use onion. If you can't get saffron, leave it out. If you are vegetarian, use vegetable broth. The one thing you do have to do is use a rice that will release the starches that make the dish sing. Arborio is available almost everywhere these days, but carnaroli is also great.

The second key to risotto is the stirring—it must be constant. That may sound like a pain, but it is the stirring that releases the starches in the rice to create the wonderful, creamy texture. You may not use all of the broth—every batch is slightly different—but once you know the technique you can adapt it endlessly. Be sure to keep the broth close; have it simmering on the burner next to or just behind the pan where you are making your risotto.

ARANCINI

2 cups leftover Saffron Risotto
  (page 116), room temperature
½ cup grated Parmesan
5 tablespoons heavy cream, divided
2 tablespoons minced fresh flat-leaf
  parsley
3 large eggs, divided

Kosher salt and freshly ground
  pepper, to taste
½ cup all-purpose flour
1½ cups breadcrumbs
Peanut, grapeseed, or canola oil,
  for frying
Warm marinara sauce, for dipping

In a large bowl, combine the Saffron Risotto, Parmesan, half the cream, parsley, and 1 of the eggs. Season with salt and pepper.

Roll about 1½ tablespoons of the risotto mixture in your palms to form a ball the size of a walnut and set aside on a baking sheet or plate. Repeat this process with the remaining risotto mixture; you should end up with 32 to 36 balls.

To arrange a breading station, set out 3 shallow baking dishes. Place the flour in the first; in the second place the remaining 2 eggs and the remaining half of cream, beating them together until smooth; and place the breadcrumbs in the third. Dip a risotto ball into the flour. Next, dip the ball into the egg mixture. Last, roll the ball in the breadcrumbs until coated. Set aside and repeat the process with the remaining risotto balls.

Transfer the balls to a baking sheet, arranging in a single layer, and store in the fridge, uncovered, for 2 to 24 hours. Preheat the oven to 200°F.

In a large sauté pan set over medium-high heat, heat ½ inch of the oil until it shimmers. Add the chilled balls, without crowding, and pan-fry them in batches for 4 to 5 minutes, turning the balls until they are evenly brown all over. Using a slotted spoon or tongs, transfer the arancini to paper towels to drain. Hold in the oven while you fry the remaining batches.

Serve right away with a bowl of the marinara sauce.

NOTE: If you want to freeze the arancini, do not pan-fry them; freeze them on a baking sheet for at least 4 hours, until solid. Then transfer them to a zip-top bag and keep them in the freezer until you're ready to pan-fry. It will take a bit longer (5 to 6 minutes) to cook them, but they keep well in the freezer for up to 3 months.

Poached Stone Fruit

SERVES 4 (WITH HALF LEFT OVER)

Poached stone fruits are great in the summer when plums, peaches, and the like are in juicy abundance. The only problem is that when they are perfectly ripe, they can go from ideal to mushy and overripe in just a day. Part of being environmentally conscious is focusing on food waste. Think of how much effort goes into growing a piece of fruit: the labor of the farmers, the water used in keeping the trees healthy, the transportation costs and environmental impact of getting them from the farm to your home. It is estimated that 72 billion pounds of food are wasted in this country every year! It can be very easy to take that bruised peach out of the fruit bowl and just toss it. But this recipe saves it, and the more we remember to find ways to use up the less-than-perfect but still edible foods in our home, the more environmentally well we become. Poaching fruits when they aren't perfect for eating out of hand honors their ripeness, and then using the leftovers to make a baked crisp makes them last all week. I use peaches here, but any stone fruits work great, including combinations, so use what you have!

1 cup granulated sugar
4 tablespoons cornstarch
12 medium peaches, pitted and halved
2 tablespoons freshly squeezed lemon juice
1 cup white wine or white grape juice

1 cinnamon stick
Whipped cream, Greek yogurt, or crème fraîche, for garnish
Toasted pumpkin seeds (see Note on page 159), for garnish

In a small bowl, mix together the sugar and the cornstarch. In a large bowl, toss the peaches with the lemon juice. Fold in the sugar mixture and transfer the sugared fruit to a Dutch oven.

Add the wine and cinnamon stick and bring to a boil over medium-high heat. Reduce the heat to medium-low and simmer for about 3 minutes, until the fruit is fork tender but still whole. Remove from the heat and let the fruit cool in its juices.

Transfer half of the peaches (12 peach halves) and juice to an airtight container and save in the fridge for a future use. Serve the remaining half of the poached fruit warm with a spoonful of the juice. Garnish with whipped cream and pumpkin seeds.

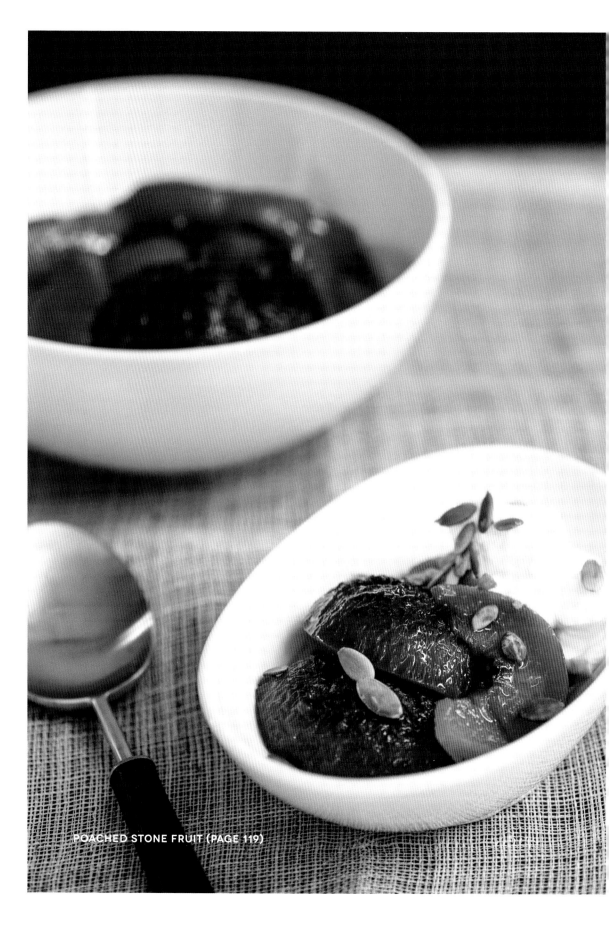

POACHED STONE FRUIT (PAGE 119)

FRUIT CRISP

SERVES 8

½ recipe Poached Stone Fruits
  (page 119)
1 cup firmly packed light brown
  sugar
1 teaspoon ground cinnamon
½ cup all-purpose flour

1 stick unsalted butter, room
  temperature
½ cup rolled oats
Whipped cream or ice cream, for
  garnish

Preheat the oven to 400°F. Grease a 9 × 13-inch baking dish.

Remove the peach halves from their juice and cut each half into 3
pieces. Arrange the pieces in the prepared baking dish; they can
overlap slightly. Pour the reserved juices over the fruit. Set aside.

In a medium bowl, combine the sugar, cinnamon, and flour until
well mixed. Using a fork or your fingers, add in the butter and mix
until you have a crumbly mixture similar in texture to large crumbs.
Add the oats and stir until well combined. Add the oat topping to
the fruit in an even layer.

Bake for 15 to 20 minutes, until the fruit is hot and the topping is
crisp. Remove the fruit crisp from the oven and set aside to cool
slightly. Serve warm, garnished with whipped cream.

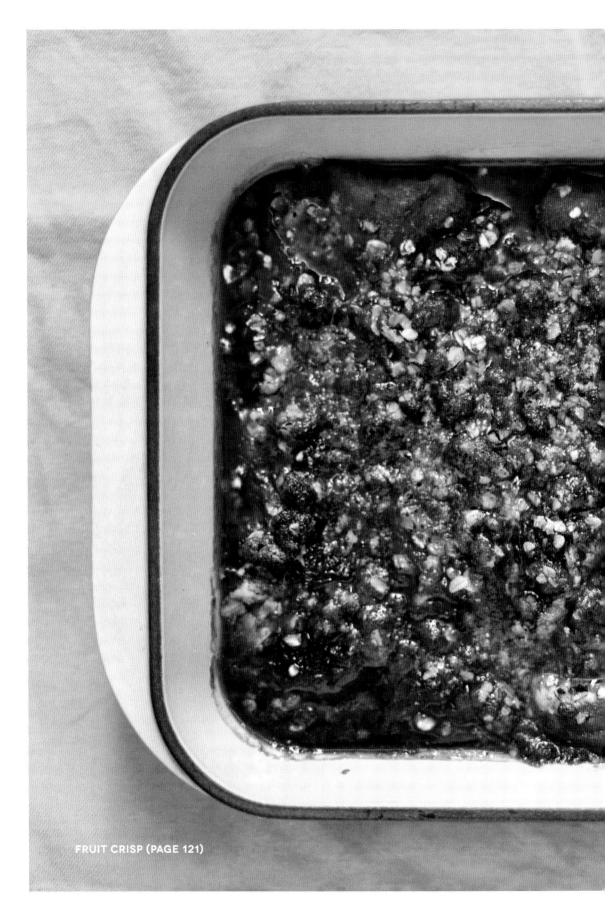

FRUIT CRISP (PAGE 121)

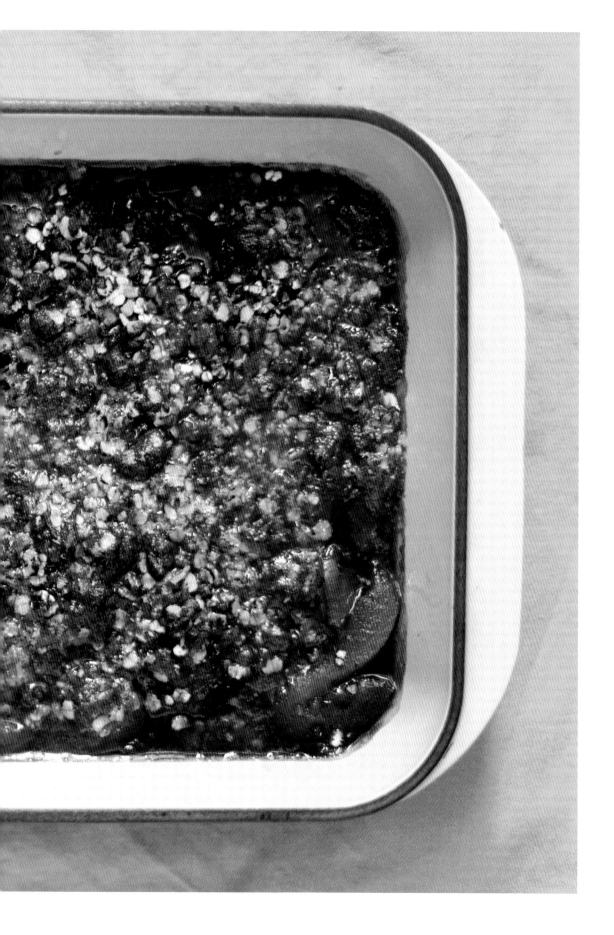

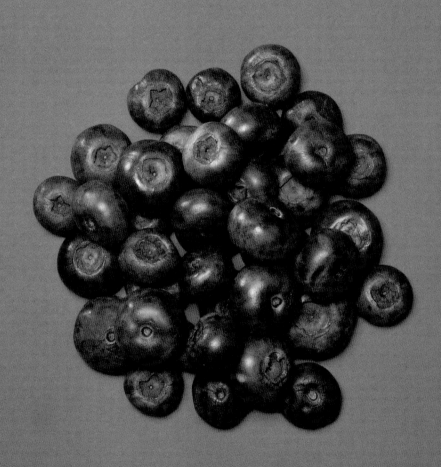

CHAPTER 5: Intellectual Wellness

INTELLECTUAL WELLNESS IS ABOUT **LEARNING**. Most people have never explored what it truly means to learn, but by doing so, they maximize the capacity of their cognitive abilities—otherwise known as brainpower. The learning process includes five basic steps: readiness, stimulus, discovery, response, and application. To illustrate this, let's use the example of learning about the intersection of cooking, eating, and your overall well-being.

Readiness means you make a conscious and deliberate commitment to reading each chapter introduction in this book. *Stimulus* involves enticing your senses at the onset of the lesson to get you excited, which is why I used beautiful, colorful photography to illustrate our tempting recipes. *Discovery* is the time that you spend actually reading and studying this book. *Response* includes your "aha" moments, such as learning for the first time that there are five steps in the learning process. Finally, *application* occurs when you actually prepare one of the recipes and enjoy the fruits of your efforts.

COOKING for your intellectual well-being means applying the five steps of the learning process. Prior to preparing the recipes in this chapter, make a firm decision to become a student of the cooking arts by reading (or rereading) this chapter introduction. A lot is being said these days about neuroplasticity, but the simplest way to think about it is that when you do thinking activities, like crossword puzzles or learning a new language, your brain reacts much like a muscle you are using and making stronger. Cooking can be like a new language, and there are certain techniques that might not be a part of your repertoire of current skills. We have included recipes in this chapter that show you some cooking techniques that require you to focus and follow specific sets of directions, which is great for neuroplasticity. Finally, apply your newfound knowledge of brainpower foods by actually preparing them!

EATING for your intellectual well-being means selecting the right combination of foods that maximize cognition or brain-power, minimize the dreaded blood-sugar crash, and support brain health. We've selected recipes in this chapter that include these very foods—low glycemic ones that keep your brain healthy and high functioning, and are less likely to cause you to crash. They help you to maintain your blood-sugar levels, which translates into a better ability to concentrate, retain information, effectively listen, and articulate your thoughts to others. Enjoy these foods prior to anything important—a job interview, a college class, a date, etc.—and perform at your peak!

Enjoy these foods prior to anything important—a job interview, a college class, a date, etc.—and perform at your peak!

Steamed Artichokes

SERVES 4

Artichokes are food for your brain. They are full of vitamin K, which can reduce neuron damage. Studies now say that vitamin K is recommended for people dealing with dementia or Alzheimer's. Artichokes can also help open up your blood vessels so that more oxygen can reach your brain. Increased oxygen in the brain can improve cognition. When you combine that with a preparation and cooking process that is very precise, you can also keep your brain working in new ways. Need more convincing? Artichokes are ridiculously delicious. Once you master the process described here, you'll find that artichokes are a very easy and welcome addition to your spring cooking.

4 artichokes (see Note)
1 lemon, halved

Meyer Lemon Dipping Sauce (recipe follows), for serving

Pour 2 inches of water into a large stockpot. Place a steamer basket or steaming insert into the pot. Set aside. Rinse the artichokes under cold running water and let dry.

To prep the artichokes, use a sharp, serrated kitchen knife to trim the stem flush with the bottom of the artichoke, being careful not to cut off any of the heart. Snap off the tough outer leaves and discard them, being careful not to prick yourself with the thorns. Rest the artichoke on its side and, using the serrated knife, slice off the top inch, cutting through all of the leaves. If there are any leaves remaining with a top, snip them off with scissors.

With the cut side of the lemon, rub the bottom, top, and any cut edges of the artichoke. Place the artichoke, bottom-side up, in the steamer basket. If any leaves are resting in the water, remove them so that the artichoke is suspended; this will prevent it from becoming waterlogged.

Repeat this process with the remaining artichokes, arranging them in the pot with some space between them so that the steam can fully surround them. Cover the pot, set it over medium-high heat, and cook until a fork easily pierces the bottom and the heart is tender, 35 to 45 minutes depending on their size.

Serve hot or cold with the Meyer Lemon Dipping Sauce.

NOTE: When shopping for artichokes, find ones that are heavy for their size, with tight, compact heads that squeak a little if you squeeze them.

Meyer Lemon Dipping Sauce

Zest and freshly squeezed juice from 1 Meyer
    lemon (see Note)
3 tablespoons Dijon mustard, plus more as
    needed
¼ teaspoon kosher salt, plus more to taste
¼ teaspoon freshly ground white pepper, plus
    more to taste
4 tablespoons minced chives, divided
¾ cup extra virgin olive oil
Honey or sugar, to taste

In the bowl of a blender or food processor,
or in a large bowl and using an immersion
blender, blend together the Meyer lemon
zest and juice, mustard, salt, pepper, and 3
tablespoons of the chives until smooth.

With the machine running, add the oil
in a small stream until all of the oil has
been incorporated and the dressing has
achieved a silky, smooth texture. Be sure to
stop the blending as soon as the dressing is
emulsified; if you process olive oil for too
long, it becomes bitter.

Taste and add salt and pepper as needed. If
the dressing isn't sharp enough, add more
of the mustard. If it's too sharp, add a bit
of honey or sugar to temper it.

Stir in the remaining 1 tablespoon of chives.
Transfer the dressing to an airtight container and store in the fridge for up to 1 week.
Bring to room temperature before using.

> **NOTE:** Meyer lemons are slightly sweeter
> and more fragrant than regular lemons. If
> you can't find them, use the juice of one regular lemon with the zest of one tangerine
> and ½ teaspoon of superfine sugar to mimic
> the floral impact of the Meyer lemon.

Chicken Consommé

Chicken soup has long been known to be good for you. It has immunity-boosting properties that will help fend off colds and help you heal if you do get stricken. But, chicken soup is rarely considered elegant. The difference between chicken soup and chicken consommé is process. Think of unfamiliar cooking techniques like this one as puzzles for your brain. Just like crossword puzzles and "brain-twister" games have been shown to positively impact brain health, when you learn a new cooking method, particularly one that is as specific as this one, you can help increase your neural plasticity—literally make your brain stronger! Consommé is a showstopper but easier than you think. It isn't difficult; it is just precise, which is why it is a good brain exercise. But more importantly, it retains all of the health benefits of its down-home chicken soup cousin, but with the benefit of a cooking process and technique that exercises your brain!

3 large egg whites
9 ounces boneless, skinless chicken thighs
½ large yellow onion, chopped
1 carrot, peeled and chopped
1 rib celery, chopped
1 plum tomato, chopped

4 cups homemade or store-bought low-sodium
    chicken stock
Kosher salt, to taste
Traditional Garnishes (recipe follows),
    for serving

In a large mixing bowl, lightly whip the egg whites until they are foamy. Put the chicken thighs in the bowl of a food processor and pulse until coarsely ground, about the consistency of chunky peanut butter. It should not be a smooth paste. Add the ground chicken to the egg whites and mix to combine. Add the onion, carrot, celery, and tomato and mix to combine.

Pour the chicken stock into a large stockpot. (Or, use any pot that is taller than it is wide; you want something narrow here. If you use a wide pot, the ingredients you are adding to clarify the soup into consommé won't come together as tightly as you need them to do their magic.) Stir in the chicken mixture until it is thoroughly mixed with the stock.

Set the pot over high heat and, with a rubber spatula or wooden spoon, stir continuously, until the mixture begins to simmer. Reduce the heat to medium-low and stop stirring, so that the solids in the stock will congeal and form the raft, a cohesive mass that floats on top of the stock. Once the raft has formed, reduce the heat to low and simmer, making sure the stock does not boil, for 45 minutes to 1 hour, until the broth is clear. If it does boil, the raft will break and the soup will be cloudy.

Meanwhile, line a colander or strainer with a coffee filter or a few layers of cheesecloth. Place it over a bowl and set it aside.

Once the broth is clear, it's time to remove it without disturbing the raft. You cannot simply remove the raft, as it will break and cloud the soup—all that work will have been for nothing! Instead, using a pair of spoons, gently make a small hole in the center of the raft, just large enough for your ladle to fit into. You want to just gently nudge open the hole. Using a ladle, slowly and carefully remove the broth, one ladle at a time, through the hole in the raft, and pour it into the prepared colander. Stop if you think the raft is beginning to break up. Repeat this process until you have removed as much broth as you can.

Discard the raft and whatever dregs of broth are left in the pot, as well anything in the strainer. Taste the consommé and add salt as needed. (Do not season with pepper.) Remove any sneaky bits of fat from the surface of the consommé by dragging a paper towel gently over the top. If you are serving it hot, you might need to put the consommé into a clean pot to reheat over medium-low heat.

Divide the garnishes evenly between 6 small bowls. Gently ladle the consommé, hot or cold, over them just before serving.

Traditional Garnishes

1 carrot, peeled
1 rib celery
2 cups water
1 teaspoon kosher salt

3 tablespoons Enoki mushroom caps
  (no stems), cut into 1-inch pieces
1 tablespoon minced chives

Using a Parisian baller, scoop the carrot into small balls, or just dice it small. Using a vegetable peeler, peel the top of the celery to remove the strings, then cut into 1½-inch-long chunks and slice each into matchsticks.

Rest a strainer in a small bowl of ice water so that the bowl of the strainer is filled with water, but no ice. Set this near your stovetop.

In a small saucepan set over medium-high heat, bring the water and salt to a boil. Add the carrot and celery and blanch for 1 minute. Immediately drop them into the prepared strainer to stop the cooking. Move the strainer around to be sure the vegetables are fully cooled. Drain the vegetables, and transfer them to a small bowl lined with paper towels to dry. The mushrooms and chives are used raw.

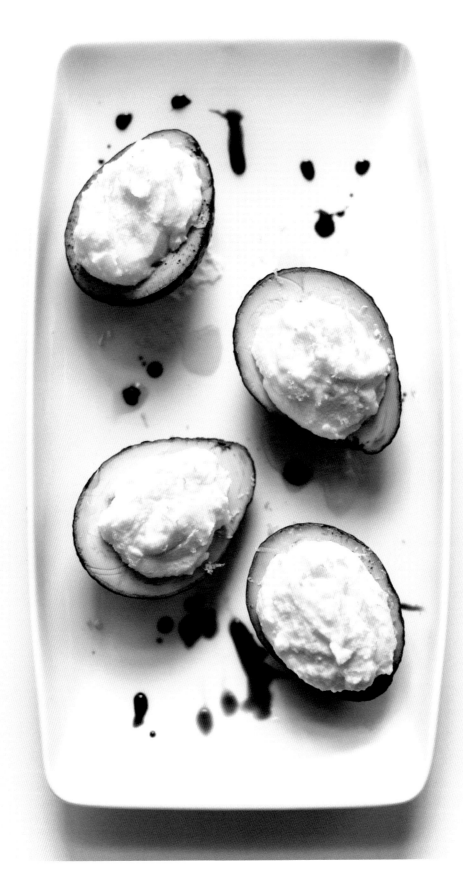

Ricotta-Stuffed Avocados

SERVES 4

Making cheese at home is less complicated than you might think, especially if you stick to fresh, easy cheeses like this ricotta. Once again, stressing new processes in your cooking positively impacts your brain health. Any new skill is great for keeping your brain working at the top of its game, and many doctors believe that exercising your mind by learning new things can help ward off dementia and Alzheimer's. Avocados are a brain booster, helping protect the brain from oxidative stress almost as well as blueberries, and are good for your blood pressure, which can keep cognitive functions working smoothly. The combination is a wonderful lunch or appetizer, and once you discover how easy it is to make your own ricotta, the gummy store-bought version will be a thing of the past.

Ricotta
2 quarts whole milk
1 cup heavy cream
3 tablespoons white vinegar
½ teaspoon kosher salt

Assembly
2 ripe avocados, halved and pitted
Kosher salt and freshly ground black pepper,
   to taste
2 tablespoons extra virgin olive oil
1 tablespoon balsamic vinegar
Zest of ½ lemon

To make the ricotta, heat the milk and cream in a medium pot set over medium heat until the surface is foamy and steamy, but not boiling; a candy or instant-read thermometer should read no more than 185°F. Remove the mixture from the heat and add the vinegar, stirring for 30 seconds to combine. Add the salt and stir for another 30 seconds. Cover the pot with a clean towel and let the mixture sit, undisturbed, at room temperature for 2 hours, until you can see that there is whey on the top and small curds have formed; it will look a bit like underwater coral.

Line a colander with several layers of cheesecloth and place it over a large bowl or suspend it over the sink. Using a slotted spoon, carefully transfer the curds to the prepared colander. Close the cheesecloth with a rubber band and let the bundle rest in the colander for 30 minutes, occasionally squeezing gently to press out the whey, until you have a fluffy and only slightly moist curd; it will look a bit like dry cottage cheese. Be sure that the colander is suspended and that the bottom is not sitting in the whey, where it can get reabsorbed.

Reserve 1 cup of the ricotta. Transfer the remaining ricotta to an airtight container and store in the fridge for a future use. It will keep for up to 4 days.

To assemble, season the avocado halves with salt and pepper. Pour ½ tablespoon of the oil and ¼ tablespoon of the balsamic vinegar into each of the 4 pit holes. Gently place ¼ cup of the reserved ricotta onto each avocado half.

Garnish with the lemon zest and serve.

White Bean Tuna Salad

SERVES 2

Tuna, especially when packed in olive oil, is full of omega-3 fatty acids, which support brain health. Radicchio is full of vitamin K, which helps limit neuron damage in the brain, and its polyphenols help to neutralize free radicals for mental quickness. The luteolin in parsley helps guard against neuron degeneration, and beans in general help stabilize glucose levels, keeping the brain well fed. So when I saw a version of this salad in *Bon Appétit* magazine, I was inspired. This salad is easy to pull together and an excellent addition to your repertoire.

1 small head radicchio
1 head endive
½ cup fresh flat-leaf parsley leaves
2 (15-ounce) cans small white navy beans, rinsed and drained
1 small English cucumber, seeded and diced medium

2 ribs celery, sliced thin
1 tablespoon red wine vinegar
3 tablespoons extra virgin olive oil
Kosher salt and freshly ground black pepper, to taste
2 (4-ounce) cans tuna packed in olive oil, drained and broken into large pieces

With a large chef's knife, halve the radicchio through the core. Remove the core from each half by making a V-shaped cut around the core. Pull off any damaged outer leaves and discard them along with the core pieces.

Cut the radicchio into 2-inch slices and put in a large mixing bowl. Separate the leaves of endive from the core and cut into 1-inch slices. Add the endive to the bowl. Add the parsley, beans, cucumber, and celery and toss to combine.

In a small bowl, mix the vinegar and oil together and pour it over the salad, tossing well. Taste and add salt and pepper as needed.

Divide the salad into two large, shallow bowls. Add the flaked tuna equally to both and serve.

Chicken Thigh Mole

SERVES 6

We could go through the brain health benefits of many of the ingredients in mole, but it would make this book significantly longer. Trust me, the combination of spices, chiles, and chocolate make this sauce terrific for your brain. But the reason I am including it here is the process. Nothing is better for developing neuroplasticity than to engage in new and precise cooking techniques. Are there nearly 30 ingredients in this recipe? Yep—but I'm not apologizing. Mole is a slow, steady process, which means it is good for your brain and even better for your belly. Once you have made it from scratch, it will become a special treat, the perfect thing to make on a cold, lazy weekend afternoon when you can focus on the process. I would never presume to develop a mole completely from scratch on my own, so I have adapted this recipe from modern Mexican cuisine master Rick Bayless. His version uses many of the same ingredients, but we have streamlined the process a bit to make it a bit easier to tackle for the home cook. Once you master this version, check out the original to take it to the next level!

6 dried ancho chiles
6 dried guajillo chiles
2 dried pasilla chiles
2½ tablespoons sesame seeds
1 teaspoon cumin seeds
½ teaspoon whole fennel seeds
½ teaspoon coriander seeds
½ teaspoon whole black peppercorns
¼ teaspoon whole cloves
½ teaspoon dried thyme
¼ teaspoon dried oregano
2 dried bay leaves, crumbled
½ tablespoon ground cinnamon
3¾ cups homemade or store-bought low-sodium chicken stock, divided

¼ cup skin-on almonds
¼ cup raw shelled cashews
¼ cup hulled pumpkin seeds
4 tablespoons canola oil, divided
2 stale corn tortillas
¼ cup dried cherries
5 cloves garlic
1 small onion, thinly sliced
1 large tomatillo, husked, rinsed, and quartered
1 small plum tomato, quartered
2 pounds boneless, skinless chicken thighs
Kosher salt, to taste
½ cup finely chopped Mexican chocolate or unsweetened baking chocolate
2 tablespoons agave syrup

Remove the stems and seeds from the ancho, guajillo, and pasilla chiles, reserving the seeds in a small bowl, and then tear the chiles into large pieces. Set the torn chiles aside in a small bowl. Reserve 2 tablespoons of the combined seeds and discard the rest. Most of the heat in chiles is in the seeds, so you want to be judicious about using them! You can save the seeds you don't use for this recipe in your freezer to add a bit of heat to soups or stews.

CONTINUED ▷

Chicken Thigh Mole

Heat a small nonstick skillet over medium-high heat. Add the reserved chile seeds, sesame seeds, cumin seeds, fennel seeds, coriander seeds, peppercorns, and cloves. Cook, gently swirling the pan to keep the spices moving, until they are lightly toasted and fragrant. Transfer the toasted spices to an electric coffee grinder. Add the thyme, oregano, bay leaves, and cinnamon and grind into a fine powder. Set aside.

Bring some water to a boil and pour it over the reserved chile pieces so they are just covered. Let them steep for 30 minutes. Drain the chiles and reserve the soaking liquid.

Working in two batches, put half of the soaked chiles, 2 tablespoons of the soaking liquid, and 2 tablespoons of the chicken stock into a blender and purée on high speed. Set a strainer over a bowl and strain each batch, discarding the skins and solids. Set the chile purée aside.

Return the skillet you used to toast the spices to medium heat. Add the almonds, cashews, and pumpkin seeds and toast for about 1 minute, swirling the pan to keep them moving, until they are lightly browned. Transfer the toasted nuts and pumpkin seeds to a large bowl.

Keeping the skillet over medium heat, add 1 tablespoon of the canola oil and heat until it shimmers. Fry the tortillas, turning just once, until golden brown, about 3 minutes. Transfer the fried tortillas to paper towels to drain. Break up them into small pieces and add them to the toasted nuts and pumpkin seeds. Add the ground spice mixture and cherries.

In a large skillet set over medium-high heat, heat another tablespoon of the canola oil until it shimmers. Add the garlic and onion and cook, stirring frequently, for 10 to 15 minutes, until the onions are caramelized. Add the tomatillo and tomato and cook, stirring frequently, until soft, 10 to 12 minutes. Add this mixture to the bowl with the spice mixture. Add 1½ cups of the stock. In a blender, working in batches, purée the mixture. Strain it through a sieve the same way you did with the chiles. Set the spiced purée aside.

In a large Dutch oven over medium-high heat, heat the remaining 2 tablespoons of oil until it shimmers. Season the chicken thighs on both sides with salt. Add the chicken to the Dutch oven and cook, turning once, for about 8 minutes, until each side is brown. Transfer the chicken to a plate.

Add the chile purée to the hot Dutch oven and cook, stirring frequently, until thickened, about 10 minutes. Add the spiced purée, blend well, and reduce the heat to medium-low. Cook, stirring frequently, for 30 minutes. Add the remaining 2 cups of stock and the chocolate and stir until the chocolate is completely melted. Reduce the heat to low and cover the Dutch oven, leaving about two-thirds of the pot uncovered to release steam. Cook, stirring frequently to prevent scorching, for about 1 hour. Add the agave syrup. Taste and add salt as needed.

Preheat the oven to 350°F. Return the chicken thighs to the Dutch oven and submerge in the mole sauce. Bake, covered, about 1 hour, or until an instant-read thermometer inserted into the center of the mixture reads 165°F. Transfer the Dutch oven to a wire rack and let it rest for 20 minutes.

Slice the thighs and serve topped with the mole sauce.

> **NOTE:** This is a terrific dish to serve with classic rice and beans, but you can also use it as a filling for tacos or serve on top of a salad if you want a lighter dish.

Steaks with Red Wine Marinade

SERVES 6

Red wine, in moderation, is great for brain health, and the iron in beef helps support myelin, for quick processing, and healthy red blood cells, which bring oxygen to the brain. This marinade can be made up to four days in advance, and the steaks can go in for as little as an hour or as long as 24.

2 heads garlic
¾ cup extra virgin olive oil, divided, plus
    more for grilling and garnish
¾ cup dry Italian red wine
¼ cup fresh marjoram, chopped
½ cup fresh flat-leaf parsley leaves, chopped,
    plus more for garnish

4 shallots, sliced
Pinch red pepper flakes
1½ teaspoons kosher salt
1 teaspoon freshly ground black pepper
6 (6-ounce) flat iron steaks

Preheat the oven to 400°F.

Slice the top ½ inch off of the garlic heads to expose the cloves. Place the heads on a sheet of heavy-duty aluminum foil, drizzle with ¼ cup of the oil, and then wrap tightly in the foil. Transfer to a small baking dish and roast for 45 minutes.

Remove the garlic from the oven, carefully open the foil, and let the garlic come to room temperature. Once cool enough to handle, squeeze the roasted cloves out of 1 head into a medium bowl and mash them into a paste. Into a separate small bowl, gently pop the cloves out of the other head, keeping them whole, and set them aside.

Add the remaining ½ cup of oil to the garlic paste. Add the wine, marjoram, parsley, shallots, red pepper flakes, salt, and pepper, mixing well until the salt has dissolved into the marinade.

Pour the marinade into a gallon-size zip-top bag. Add the steaks, press out as much air as you can, and seal the bag. Smoosh the steaks around in the marinade until they are well coated. Transfer the bag to the fridge and let the steaks marinate for at least 1 hour or as long as 22 hours. Don't let the steaks stay in the marinade longer than 24 hours or it will begin to break down the meat, making the steaks mushy when cooked.

Remove the bag from the fridge and let rest at room temperature for 2 hours. Meanwhile, prepare a grill. Right before cooking, remove the steaks from the marinade and pat dry with paper towels. Discard the marinade. Lightly oil the steaks on both sides.

Set the steaks on the grill over direct heat and cook for about 3 minutes on each side, or until an instant-read thermometer inserted into the thickest part of the meat registers 130°F for medium rare. (You can also cook them in an oiled grill pan set over high heat for the same length of time.)

Transfer the steaks to plates. Drizzle a bit of olive oil over them and divide the reserved whole roasted garlic cloves among the steaks. Garnish with the parsley and serve.

Eggs Poached in Red Wine

SERVES 2

I love this particular use for red wine. The wine, with all of its resveratrol and antioxidants, is wonderful for brain health by combating the negative effects of free radicals and positively impacting glucose metabolization. Cooking eggs, usually something you do by rote, now becomes a completely new skill and a bit of a brain exerciser. But more importantly, this recipe takes eggs out of breakfast and into elegant dinner territory.

4 ounces pancetta, cubed
2 tablespoons extra virgin olive oil, divided
1 small carrot, peeled and diced
2 shallots, minced
1 rib celery, chopped
1 sprig fresh thyme
1 (750-mL) bottle full-bodied red wine,
    such as a cabernet or shiraz

4 large eggs, room temperature
1 tablespoon unsalted butter, softened
1 tablespoon all-purpose flour
2 large slices country or sourdough bread
1 clove garlic, halved
Kosher salt and freshly ground black pepper,
    to taste

In a large, wide skillet set over medium-high heat, sauté the pancetta until it is crispy and its fat has rendered. Transfer the pancetta to a plate lined with paper towels to drain, and set aside. Add 1 tablespoon of the oil to the fat in the pan. Add the carrot, shallots, celery, and thyme and sauté until the shallots are just translucent and lightly browned. Add the red wine and simmer until it has reduced by half, then remove it from the heat.

While the sauce is reducing, crack the eggs into 4 small bowls and set aside. In a separate small bowl, blend the butter and flour into a smooth paste and set aside. This is called a beurre manié, and it is a wonderful thickener for all sorts of sauces, including gravy; always use equal amounts of butter and flour.

Strain the wine sauce and discard the solids. Return it to the pan, set over medium-low heat, and bring it back to a gentle simmer.

Toast the bread. While it is still hot, rub the toast with the cut side of the garlic. Drizzle the remaining 1 tablespoon of oil over the toast and place each piece on a plate.

Slowly whisk the beurre manié into the wine sauce, and continue whisking constantly until the sauce has thickened slightly. Taste and add salt and pepper as needed. Quickly slip the eggs, one at a time, from their bowls into the wine sauce, on opposite sides of the pan, making sure that they don't touch. Cook, gently spooning some of the wine sauce over the tops of the eggs so that they cook completely, for about 2 minutes. The whites should be fully set, and the yolks should be warm but still runny.

Using a slotted spoon, add 2 eggs to each piece of toast. Add a spoonful of the wine sauce over each serving. Garnish with the crispy pancetta and serve.

Rib Chops with Pomegranate Marinade

SERVES 6

Antioxidants are really important for brain health. They help combat the harmful effects of free radicals, to which brain cells are particularly susceptible. The benefit of the antioxidants in pomegranates is well documented, and their tart sweetness is a wonderful, unexpected pairing for pork. I never thought of cooking with pomegranates in savory dishes until I saw a version of this recipe on *Cooking with Books*. While I love the health benefits of pomegranates, I always thought that apples were the best fruit to pair with pork chops! But the brightness of the pomegranate made a believer out of me. Marinate the chops either the night before or the morning of the day you want to cook them, and they will be ready to go in time for dinner.

1½ cups pomegranate juice

2 tablespoons pomegranate molasses

5 tablespoons extra virgin olive oil, divided, plus more for brushing

3 tablespoons balsamic vinegar

6 tablespoons firmly packed light brown sugar

3 teaspoons fine sea salt, plus more for serving

1½ teaspoons freshly ground black pepper

6 (6-ounce) bone-in pork rib chops

2 tablespoons chopped fresh flat-leaf parsley, for garnish

In a small saucepan set over low heat, warm the pomegranate juice, the pomegranate molasses, 4 tablespoons of the oil, the vinegar, the sugar, the salt, and the pepper, stirring until the mixture is warmed but not hot and the sugar and molasses are melted and fully mixed in.

Pour the marinade into a gallon-size zip-top bag and add the pork chops. Press out as much air as possible before sealing the bag. Smoosh the chops around in the bag until they are well coated. Transfer the bag to the fridge and let the chops marinate for at least 8 hours or as long as 24 hours. Don't let the chops marinate longer than 24 hours, as the acid in the marinade will break down the pork too much, giving it a mushy texture when cooked.

Heat a cast-iron or stainless steel skillet over medium-high heat, and add the remaining 1 tablespoon of oil. Remove the chops from the marinade and dry both sides well with paper towels. Lightly oil both sides of the chops. Reserve the marinade and set aside. Add the chops to the skillet and sear for 3 to 5 minutes per side, until both sides are nicely browned. Pour the reserved marinade into the skillet, and bring it to a boil. Cook for 1 minute, and then reduce the heat to low and simmer, turning the chops once, for about 5 more minutes, until the pork is cooked through and an instant-read thermometer inserted into the thickest part of the meat reads 145°F.

Transfer the pork from the skillet to a platter and let rest for 10 minutes. Increase the heat to medium-high and bring the marinade back to a boil. Let it reduce until the glaze has the approximate consistency of heavy cream.

Serve the pork with the glaze spooned over, sprinkled lightly with salt and garnished with parsley.

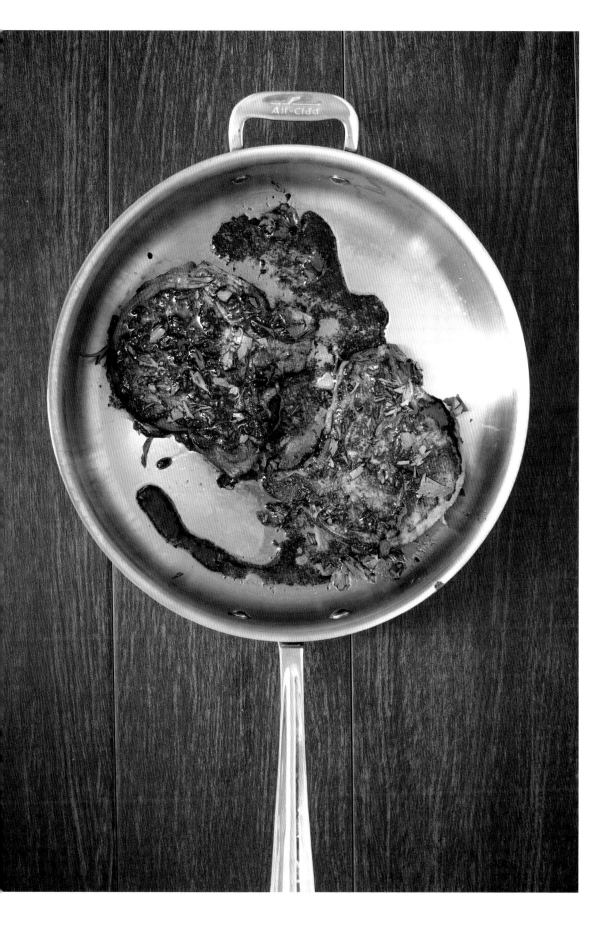

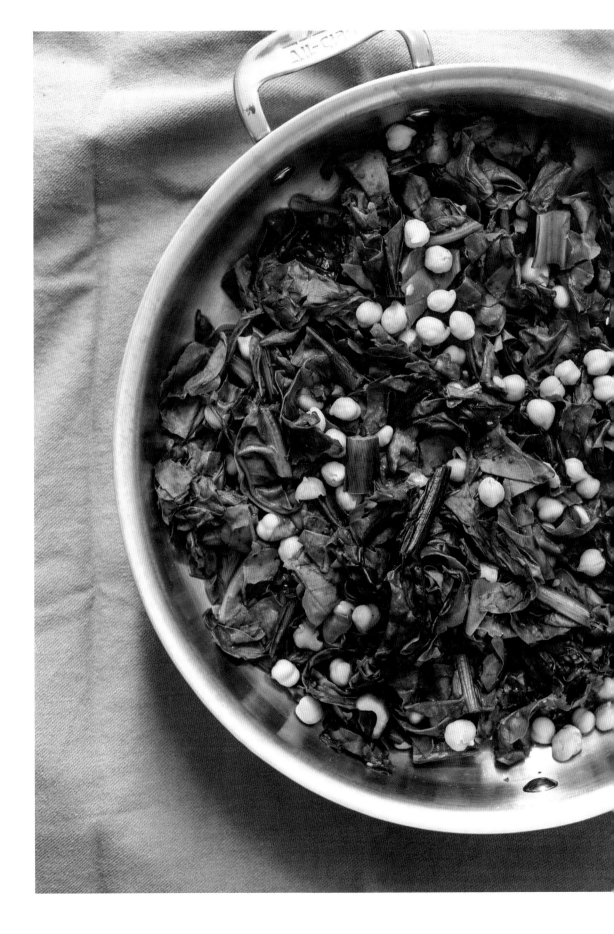

Swiss Chard and Chickpeas

SERVES 2 AS AN ENTRÉE OR 4 AS A SIDE

Leafy green vegetables are a superfood for a reason, and their benefits for brain health are well documented. The lutein they contain can help prevent cognitive decline. Adding protein-packed chickpeas makes this a wonderful entrée when served over brown rice.

2 bunches Swiss chard
2 tablespoons extra virgin olive oil, plus more for garnish
1 (15-ounce) can chickpeas, drained and rinsed
1 teaspoon Worcestershire sauce
1 tablespoon white balsamic or white wine vinegar

½ cup homemade or store-bought low-sodium chicken stock
Pinch red pepper flakes (optional)
Kosher salt and freshly ground black pepper, to taste

Separate the stems from the leaves of the chard, cut the stems into ½-inch slices, and tear the leaves into 1½-inch pieces. Set the prepped chard aside.

In a large skillet set over medium-high heat, heat the oil until it shimmers. Add the chickpeas and sauté until they are slightly golden and crispy. Add the chard stems and cook for 1 minute. Sprinkle in the Worcestershire sauce and vinegar and cook until the liquid is nearly evaporated.

Add the chard leaves and gently combine with the stems and chickpeas. Add the chicken stock and red pepper flakes, if using. Continue to sauté until the leaves are tender and the stock is mostly gone, 5 to 6 minutes. Taste and add salt and pepper as needed.

Finish with a drizzle of the oil and serve hot.

Roasted Wild Mushrooms with Braised Pistachios

I have always loved nuts for their health benefits but never thought of them as much more than a healthy snack or a crunchy addition to sweets. Then I saw a recipe from Justin Aprahamian for braised pistachios that blew my mind. Turns out, braising pistachio nuts gives them a wonderful taste and texture, much like a bean. Combining them with meaty roasted mushrooms makes for an unusual side dish that packs a flavor punch, in addition to the health benefits. Mushrooms are good for brain and nerve health because they can help boost nerve growth factor, which helps build gray matter in the brain. Pistachios are rich in vitamin B6, which supports myelin development, and are also a good source of vitamin K.

Braised Pistachios
3 tablespoons extra virgin olive oil
3 shallots, sliced
3 cups shelled pistachios
3 tablespoons white wine vinegar
1 sprig fresh thyme
4 cups homemade or store-bought
   low-sodium chicken stock, plus more
   as needed
Kosher salt and freshly ground black
   pepper, to taste

Roasted Mushrooms
3 pounds mixed fresh mushrooms, such as
   cremini, chanterelle, and shiitake, cleaned
   (see Note on page 145)
⅓ cup extra virgin olive oil
1 shallot, minced
8 sprigs fresh thyme
Zest and freshly squeezed juice of 1 lemon
1 teaspoon kosher salt, plus more to taste
½ teaspoon freshly ground black pepper,
   plus more to taste
3 tablespoons chopped fresh flat-leaf parsley
2 tablespoons minced chives, for garnish

To make the braised pistachios, in a medium sauté pan set over medium heat, heat the oil until it shimmers. Add the shallots and cook for about 5 minutes, until they are translucent and golden brown.

Add the pistachios and stir to coat well. Add the vinegar and cook until nearly all of the liquid is gone. Add the thyme and stock and bring the mixture to a gentle boil. Reduce the heat to low and simmer, stirring occasionally and making sure that the stock is being slowly absorbed but the pan doesn't go dry, for about 1 hour, until the pistachios are soft but not mushy, like a firm bean, and the liquid just creates a glaze over the cooked nuts. If the liquid is disappearing too quickly, add a bit more stock or water. Taste and add salt and pepper as needed. Set aside.

To make the roasted mushrooms, preheat the oven to 400°F. Line a large baking sheet with aluminum foil and set aside. Destem the mushrooms. Then, halve the small mushrooms and quarter the large ones. Transfer the prepped mushrooms to a large bowl.

In a small bowl, combine the oil, shallot, thyme, lemon zest and juice, salt, and pepper, mixing well. Pour the mixture over the mushrooms and stir until the mushrooms are evenly coated.

Arrange the mushrooms on the prepared pan in a single layer so that there is plenty of space between each mushroom and no crowding. Use 2 pans if necessary. This is a good idea when roasting any vegetable; if the pieces touch, they will steam instead of roast.

Roast the mushrooms for about 15 minutes. Check to see if they have released their liquid. All mushrooms are different, so you might have a lot of liquid or very little. Regardless, juices are the enemy of roasting, so remove the pan from the oven and pour off the juices over a strainer (to catch any mushrooms that fall). Return the mushrooms to the pan, stir them with a large spatula, and again arrange them to prevent crowding.

Continue roasting for 20 minutes, until the mushrooms are well browned but still tender. If the mushrooms are not yet done, roast for another 5 to 10 minutes, checking frequently to avoid making mushroom jerky. After about 15 minutes of the 20-minute cook time, return the pistachios to medium-low heat and let them warm up.

Remove the mushrooms from the oven and discard the thyme sprigs. Transfer the mushrooms to a bowl and toss with the parsley and the braised pistachios. Taste and add salt and pepper as needed. Garnish with the chopped chives and serve hot.

NOTE: The braised pistachios will keep up to 3 days in an airtight container in the fridge.

To wash mushrooms, if they are not very dirty, wipe them clean with a paper towel. If they have a lot of grit on them, rinse them quickly in cold water and dry immediately. This may seem like a lot of work, but mushrooms require fairly precise cleaning. Most of them are grown in pasteurized manure—which won't poison you but is not pleasant to eat—and they are like little sponges that soak up water if not cleaned and dried carefully, which will give them a mushy texture when cooked.

Lentil Salad

Lentils are a great source of folate, which boosts brainpower and decreases the levels of amino acids that can negatively impact brain function. It is important to use whole lentils here; the small green du Puy lentils or the light-brown Italian lentils are best. Don't use the red, yellow, or green split lentils, as they will turn to mush! This makes a wonderful side dish but can also be an elegant luncheon salad with a piece of seared tuna or salmon on top.

1½ cups dried du Puy lentils
½ cup finely minced celery
1 tablespoon finely minced shallot
1 tablespoon sherry vinegar
3 tablespoons extra virgin olive oil
½ teaspoon kosher salt, plus more to taste

¼ teaspoon freshly ground black pepper, plus more to taste
2 tablespoons chopped fresh flat-leaf parsley
1½ tablespoons chopped fresh basil
2 tablespoons chopped chives
Grated Parmesan, for garnish

Bring a medium pot of salted water to a boil over medium-high heat and add the lentils, cooking as you would al dente pasta: 10 to 15 minutes, until cooked but still firm to the tooth. Drain the lentils in a strainer.

Put the drained lentils, celery, and shallot in a medium bowl and toss to combine. Add the vinegar, oil, salt, and pepper, mixing well. Taste and add salt and pepper as needed. Stir in the parsley, basil, and chives. Garnish with the grated Parmesan.

Serve at room temperature.

> **NOTE:** You can hold this salad at room temperature for up to six hours before serving. If you want to make it the day before, be sure to let the dish sit at room temperature for at least an hour before you serve it.

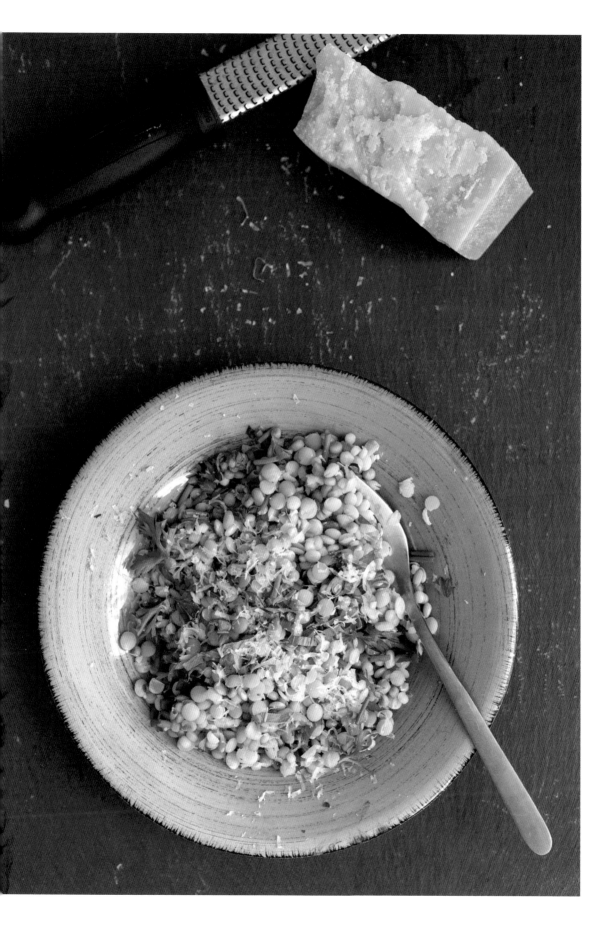

Kasha Pilaf

SERVES 4 AS A SIDE

Kasha, also known as toasted buckwheat groats, is a terrific superfood: very high in protein, easily digested, and full of the amino acids known to reduce hypertension and keep oxygen flowing freely to your brain. It has a wonderful nutty flavor, and this simple pilaf goes with any meat or fish you care to pair with it. The cooking technique is a little unusual—coating the grains with egg white first to prep them, and then simmering for tenderness—but learning this unique new skill will help keep your brain on its toes!

2 large egg whites
½ cup kasha
2 teaspoons canola oil
1 rib celery, sliced thin
1 small yellow onion, coarsely chopped

1 cup homemade or store-bought low-sodium chicken stock or broth
Freshly ground black pepper, to taste
Kosher salt, to taste (optional)
½ cup toasted slivered almonds (see Note on page 159)

In a small bowl, slightly beat the egg whites, and then spoon off about 1 teaspoon and discard. Add the kasha and toss with the whites until completely covered.

Heat a large nonstick skillet over medium heat until a hand placed about 2 inches over the surface feels the heat radiating from the pan, then add the kasha mixture. Cook, stirring frequently, until each grain is separate and dry, about 3 minutes.

Transfer the dry kasha to a clean medium bowl. In the same skillet, still over medium heat, heat the oil until it shimmers. Add the celery and onion and sauté for few minutes, until the onion begins to soften and brown. Add the kasha and stir to combine.

Add the chicken stock, reduce the heat to medium-low, and simmer, covered, for about 15 minutes, or until the kasha is tender but not mushy. Taste and add salt and pepper as needed. Using a fork to prevent clumping, toss the almonds into the kasha. Transfer to a serving bowl and serve hot.

Lemon–Blueberry Pavlova with Dark Chocolate

Blueberries are one of the healthiest superfoods all around and are especially good in helping to reverse oxidative stress in the brain. By using fresh blueberries for half of this recipe, you keep all of the benefits. In addition to being good friends with blueberry, flavor wise, lemon juice has potassium, which is beneficial for brain and nerve health. And many people have never made meringue before, which gives us a great technique to exercise a new part of our brains. I always loved blueberry and lemon together, usually in the form of a blueberry muffin with lemon glaze! I first tasted this different combination at Stacey's house, and it blew my mind. She said it was a version of a dessert she had eaten in Australia. We added the dark chocolate, since it is full of antioxidants. Plus they are all extra yummy together!

Meringue
1 cup superfine sugar (see Note on page 151)
1 tablespoon cornstarch
2 large egg whites, room temperature
2 tablespoons cold water
1 teaspoon distilled white vinegar

Lemon Curd
1 large whole egg
1 large egg yolk
5 tablespoons granulated sugar
Pinch kosher salt
½ tablespoon lemon zest
¼ cup freshly squeezed lemon juice

2½ tablespoons unsalted butter, diced
½ teaspoon fresh tarragon, finely minced

Blueberry Compote
1 pint fresh blueberries, divided
1 cup blueberry preserves
1 tablespoon white wine
1 tablespoon granulated sugar
Pinch kosher salt

Assembly
1 cup whipping cream
1 teaspoon superfine sugar
1 (4-ounce) dark chocolate bar, shaved with
   a vegetable peeler into curls

Preheat the oven to 300°F. Trace a 7-inch circle on a piece of parchment paper, flip it over, and place it on a baking sheet. Set aside.

To make the meringue, in a small bowl whisk together the superfine sugar and cornstarch. In the bowl of a stand mixer fitted with the whisk attachment, beat the egg whites on low speed until the whites get foamy, then increase the speed to medium-high and let the mixer run until soft peaks form. Increase the speed to high and, with the machine still running, add the water and beat to soft peaks again. Add the sugar mixture, 1 tablespoon at a time, and continue beating. After you add the last of the sugar mixture, beat for 1 minute more. Add the vinegar and beat, still on medium-high speed, until stiff, glossy peaks form, about 5 minutes.

CONTINUED ▷

Lemon–Blueberry Pavlova with Dark Chocolate

CONTINUED

Transfer the meringue to the prepared baking sheet, spreading evenly within the circle you drew on the parchment paper. Bake for 45 minutes. Turn the oven off, prop the door open, and let the meringue cool in the oven for 1 hour. Wash and dry the mixer bowl and put in the fridge to chill.

To make the lemon curd, in a small bowl whisk together the egg, yolk, and sugar until completely combined. Add in the salt, lemon zest and juice, butter, and tarragon, whisking again to combine. Transfer the mixture to a medium, heavy-bottomed pan set over medium-low heat. Cook, whisking constantly as the butter emulsifies into the egg, for about 3 minutes, or until the mixture comes together and resembles a thick, glossy pudding. You want to really watch the heat here; if it's too hot, the eggs could scramble or the butter could break.

As soon as you see that thickness, remove the pan from the heat and transfer the curd to a bowl to stop the cooking. If you don't, the curd will be too firm. Press a sheet of plastic wrap directly on top of the curd to prevent a skin from forming, and store it in the fridge until ready to use.

To make the blueberry compote, in a small saucepan heat ½ pint of the fresh blueberries over medium-high heat. Add the blueberry preserves, white wine, sugar, and salt, stirring to combine. Cook, stirring constantly, for 3 to 4 minutes, until the fresh blueberries have popped. Remove the pan from the heat and fold in the remaining ½ pint fresh blueberries. Transfer to an airtight container and store in the fridge until ready to use.

To assemble, in the chilled mixer bowl, whip the cream with the sugar until soft peaks form and set aside. Peel the parchment off the meringue and transfer it to a serving dish, flipping it over so the crunchy top is on the bottom and the soft underside is exposed. Spread the lemon curd over the meringue and top with 1 cup of the blueberry compote. (The remaining compote will last up to 1 week in the fridge and is great on pancakes or French toast!) Spread the whipped cream in generous swirls over the top and garnish with the dark chocolate.

Cut into wedges like a pie and serve.

NOTE: The lemon curd ingredients can be multiplied if you want to make extra, which will last up to 1 week in the fridge. If you don't love lemon, you can use any other citrus for this curd, so feel free to try tangerine, blood orange, grapefruit, or Key lime to mix things up a bit. The tarragon brings a wonderful, subtle anise flavor that brightens this dessert, but you can substitute thyme, lavender, or basil for different flavors—or leave it out altogether.

Superfine sugar shouldn't be confused with confectioners' sugar (or powdered sugar); it is just a finer grain of granulated sugar. You want to use it here because it will dissolve more easily in the egg whites than granulated sugar would. It can be a useful thing to keep in your pantry, but be careful: because of its texture, it is sweeter than regular granulated sugar, and they cannot be used interchangeably.

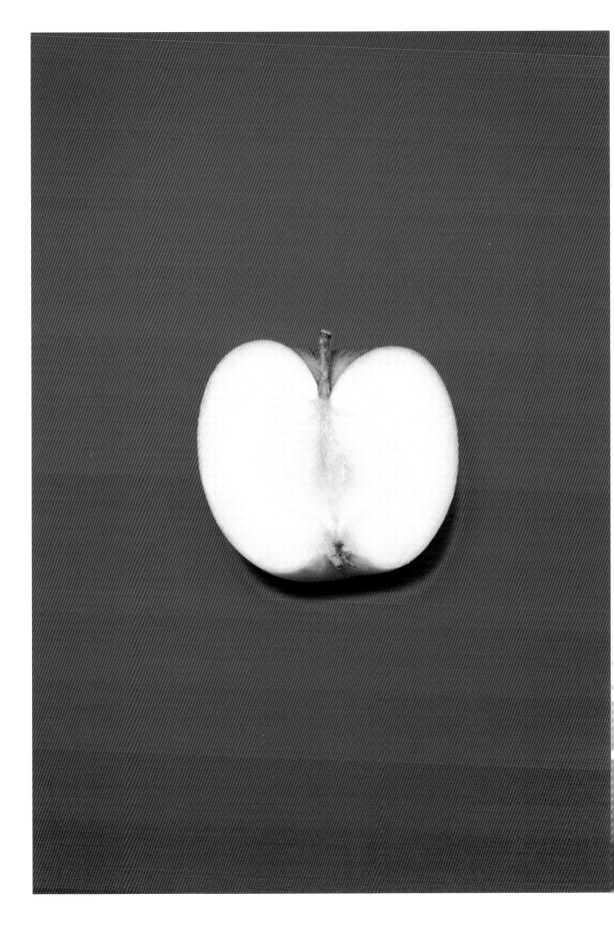

CHAPTER 6: Nutritional Wellness

NUTRITIONAL WELLNESS IS ABOUT **EATING**. It is about consuming those foods that can enhance the quality of your work and play. It is also about eating to support how you'd like to look and feel. Ultimately, and according to the best available science, it really boils down to eating foods that are high quality *and* lower in calories. Maintaining your nutritional well-being means making one of two choices: Are you eating the number of calories your body needs to maintain your current weight and health? Or, are you choosing to eat more or less, and why? If you are choosing to eat more because you are currently underweight or because you are in a period of intense physical activity that requires more fuel, eating larger portions of these good-for-you balanced foods will allow you to do that in a healthful way. If you are attempting to operate at a calorie deficit, eating less than you need to sustain your level of activity because you would like to lose some weight, you will find that these recipes allow you to feel satiated and content in the knowledge that what you are eating is good for you. Contrary to popular culture, the only "bad" foods are those that are moldy, spoiled, and allergy triggering—and suggesting otherwise can perpetuate eating disorders. You'll see that the recipes in this chapter are rich in quality ingredients, including muscle-building lean proteins, energy-providing whole grains, antioxidant-filled fruits and vegetables, and healthy, sustainable fats.

The only "bad" foods are those that are moldy, spoiled, and allergy triggering— and suggesting otherwise can perpetuate eating disorders.

COOKING for your nutritional well-being is a very satisfying proposition! It means tasting the ingredients while preparing your recipes. A burden to some, but doing so will ensure that things are as they should be, from start to finish. Sampling your good efforts along the way has several benefits. Of course, the obvious advantage is ensuring that the taste is to your liking. Additionally, it allows you to check the consistency, allowing for modifications as needed. Finally, if the cook is calorie conscious, food tasting during meal preparation amounts to healthy and purposeful snacking—making it easier to eat less at mealtime.

EATING for your nutritional well-being is about supporting the other dimensions of wellness. For example, if you are eating dinner the night before a physically active day, then consider my scrumptious and energy-yielding starches and grains. Trying to kick a late-night eating habit? My lean protein entrées will keep you satisfied longer, so that your hunger doesn't return before bedtime. Are you on a healthy eating program but have some social obligations? Why not suggest that, instead of a restaurant meal, your friends or family come to your house for a homemade, guilt-free dinner, including a healthy dessert? This chapter is loaded with foods of the highest quality that allow for relatively easy portion control *if* that happens to be your goal. Quality? Quantity? The choices are yours.

The recipes in this chapter are rich in quality ingredients, including muscle-building lean proteins, energy-providing whole grains, antioxidant-filled fruits and vegetables, and healthy, sustainable fats.

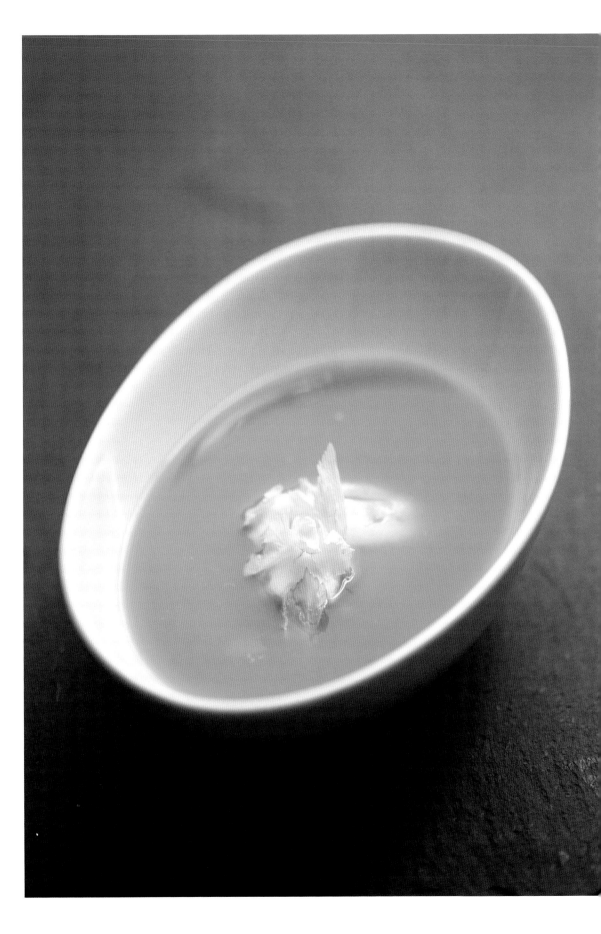

Chilled Pea Soup

SERVES 4 TO 6 AS A STARTER

A vegetable soup can be an elegant beginning to a meal, in addition to being more filling than a light salad. When you are watching what you eat, one of the most important things for progress is to not feel deprived. This soup, while low in calories, is full of bright, exciting flavors and feels like an indulgence.

1 pound high-quality frozen petite green peas
Kosher salt and freshly ground black pepper,
   to taste

Full-fat Greek yogurt or crème fraîche,
   for serving
2 tablespoons celery leaves (see Note),
   for garnish

Place the peas, still frozen, in a blender or the bowl of a food processor. Add cold water until it just reaches the top layer of peas. Do not cover them; the peas should be poking their little heads out of the water.

Purée on high speed for 2 minutes, until the texture is as smooth as possible. Strain through a fine-mesh strainer or chinois, pressing to remove all of the liquid. Taste and add salt and pepper as needed. Transfer to a covered container and store in the fridge until ready to serve.

To serve, portion into bowls. Top each portion of soup with a dollop of yogurt and add a couple of celery leaves. Serve cold.

NOTE: Celery leaves are the pale-yellow leaves on the inside of a heart of celery. While many people throw these away, they can actually contain five times as much nutritional value as the celery ribs! The tender inner leaves have wonderful celery flavor, with a bit of punch, and can be a terrific substitute for parsley. Add them to salads, chop and stir into soups, or use them to garnish anything you like!

Bresaola-Wrapped Asparagus Spears

SERVES 4

Bresaola is a cured beef, similar in texture to prosciutto but much leaner. Pairing it with gently steamed asparagus spears creates a dish that is all lean protein and healthy vegetables—the kind of appetizer that helps people who are watching what they eat feel like they are indulging without hitting the dip bowl!

16 spears thick asparagus, trimmed to about 4 inches
1 tablespoon extra virgin olive oil

Kosher salt and freshly ground black pepper, to taste
16 slices bresaola

Fill a large bowl with ice cubes and cold water. Set near your stovetop.

Fill a large pot fitted with a steamer basket with 2 inches of water. Bring to a boil over high heat. Place the asparagus in the basket and steam, covered, for 5 minutes, until the asparagus is crisp-tender, no longer raw but retaining a toothsome bite. Immediately submerge the asparagus in the ice bath to stop the cooking.

Once the asparagus spears are fully cooled, transfer them to a plate lined with paper towels and pat them dry. Transfer them to a shallow bowl. Drizzle the olive oil over them and toss to coat. Taste and add salt and pepper as needed.

Wrap each spear in a slice of the bresaola and serve at room temperature.

Healthy Crunch Salad

SERVES 12

When finding nutritional balance, one of the most difficult battles is getting your healthy carbs in without overindulging. Carbs, by nature, are calorie heavy; it's why they do such a great job of giving you energy. But, while you want and need the fiber and nutrients they provide, it is easy to overdo it on the caloric side. This salad is a fantastic way to get your whole grains, with good protein from beans and nuts and bulk from vegetables— you can eat a generous portion and stay on track. The key to this salad is texture. The riced cauliflower mimics the size and texture of the grains. A great way to reduce the carbs in a dish is to match the volume of carbs (rice, pasta, grains) one-for-one with a vegetable or legume. Many salad bars now stock a variety of cooked grains, and I often just pick them up there. There are also some good frozen versions available.

2 cups cooked mixed whole grains, such as black and red quinoa, farro, bulgur, and/or brown rice

1 cup cooked lentils, chickpeas, or the bean of your choice

½ cup shredded carrot

¼ cup toasted sunflower seeds (see Note)

2 cups riced raw cauliflower (see Note on page 109)

3 tablespoons chopped fresh flat-leaf parsley

4 tablespoons red wine vinegar

½ cup extra virgin olive oil or pumpkin seed oil

Kosher salt and freshly ground black pepper, to taste

In a large bowl, combine the cooked grains, lentils, carrot, sunflower seeds, cauliflower, and parsley, mixing well. Dress with the oil and vinegar and stir to combine, then taste and add salt and pepper as needed. Serve right away. This will keep up to 5 days in the fridge in an airtight container.

> **NOTE:** To toast any nut or seed, heat a medium nonstick skillet over medium-high heat, and swirl the pan constantly until the nuts are deepened or light golden in color and begin to give off a nutty fragrance.

Halibut with Lemon–Caper Salsa

SERVES 4

Fish is such a wonderful addition to a healthy diet; it's quick to cook, very good for you, and open to endless creativity. We've paired this light, flaky fish with a powerful salsa packed with flavor. This salsa is great with any fish but also with chicken and even on steaks!

4 (6-ounce) halibut fillets, skin removed
1 tablespoon grapeseed oil

Lemon–Caper Salsa (recipe follows),
   for serving

Preheat the oven to 400°F.

In a large nonstick, ovenproof skillet set over high heat, heat the grapeseed oil until it shimmers. Add the fillets and cook for 1 to 2 minutes, until a golden-brown crust has formed. Flip the fillets and cook for 1 minute more. Transfer the skillet to the oven and cook for 10 minutes, or until the flesh is opaque and just firm under light pressure.

Spoon salsa onto each of 4 plates. Add a fillet to each and serve right away.

Lemon–Caper Salsa

2 medium lemons
3 tablespoons finely chopped red onion
2 tablespoons Dijon mustard
2 tablespoons drained capers, finely chopped
1 tablespoon finely chopped chives

2 tablespoons finely chopped fresh flat-leaf
   parsley
½ teaspoon fine sea salt
½ teaspoon superfine sugar
¼ cup extra virgin olive oil

Supreme the lemons by completely peeling them to reveal the flesh, then carefully removing the whole segments from in between the membrane. Do this over a bowl to catch the juices, and then squeeze the separate membranes into the bowl as well to get as much juice as possible.

Add the onion, mustard, capers, chives, parsley, salt, and sugar to the bowl of lemon juice and supremes, and stir well. Add the olive oil and gently blend to combine.

Transfer the salsa to an airtight container and let rest at room temperature until serving, or store in the fridge for up to 5 days. Let it sit at room temperature for at least 30 minutes before using.

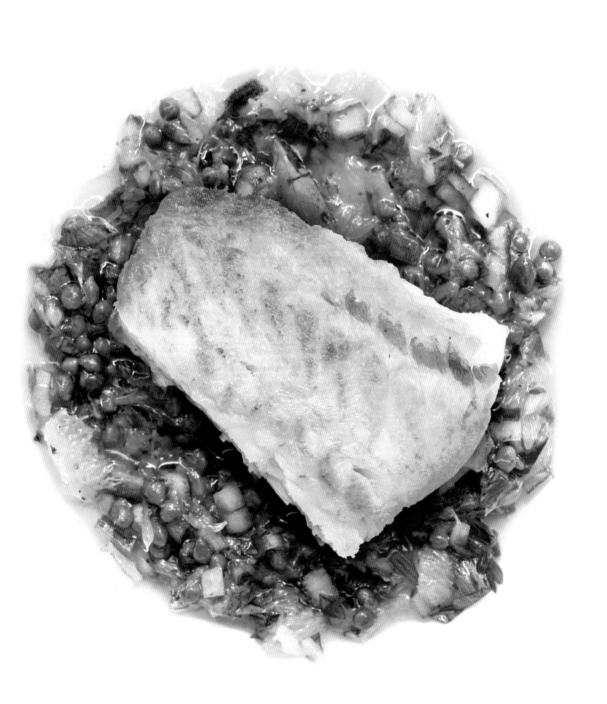

Baked Chicken with Homemade Barbecue Sauce

SERVES 4

The flavors of barbecue are often associated with fatty meats and decadence. And while ribs and brisket certainly have their place, we know that just because you are being careful about your diet doesn't mean you don't want your barbecue fix! Most bottled sauces are full of sugar and preservatives, so I developed this one, with a little Asian influence, that does double duty: it gives you guilt-free barbecue flavor, and it helps keep those notoriously fussy chicken breasts moist throughout the cooking process. Feel free to use this sauce and method with pork chops as well.

Barbecue Sauce
2 tablespoons extra virgin olive oil
⅓ cup homemade or store-bought low-sodium
   chicken stock
2 tablespoons tomato paste
1 tablespoon freshly squeezed lime juice
1 tablespoon honey
2 tablespoons tamari or soy sauce

1 teaspoon minced garlic
1 teaspoon minced fresh ginger
Pinch red pepper flakes
Pinch five-spice powder

Chicken
4 (6-ounce) boneless, skinless chicken breasts
1 tablespoon grapeseed oil

To make the barbecue sauce, combine all of the ingredients in a gallon-size zip-top bag.

To start the chicken, add the breasts to the bag of sauce, press out as much air as possible before sealing, then smoosh the chicken around in the sauce to coat everything evenly. Transfer the bag to the fridge and let the chicken marinate for at least 2 hours or as long as overnight.

Preheat the oven to 400°F.

Remove the chicken from the barbecue sauce. Reserve the barbecue sauce and pat the chicken dry with paper towels.

In a large nonstick, ovenproof skillet set over high heat, heat the oil until it shimmers. Add the chicken and cook on one side for 2 minutes, until a golden-brown crust has formed. Flip the breasts and cook for another 2 minutes. Transfer the breasts to a plate.

Pour the reserved sauce into the skillet and bring to a boil. Boil for 2 minutes, then return the chicken breasts to the skillet, being sure to turn them over in the sauce to coat them.

Transfer the skillet to the oven and bake for 12 to 15 minutes, until an instant-read thermometer registers 165°F when inserted into the thickest part of the breasts.

Remove the breasts from the sauce and let rest for 5 minutes. Serve with the sauce on the side.

Adobo Flank Steak

SERVES 4

Flank steak is a great source of lean protein, a terrific option for when you are craving beef. Even if you are cooking for only one or two people, try this recipe. The leftovers are perfect on a salad and make great sandwiches, tacos, or fajitas the next day!

2 teaspoons kosher salt
2 teaspoons freshly ground black pepper
1 teaspoon sweet paprika
2 teaspoons dried oregano
3–4 cloves garlic

2 tablespoons freshly squeezed lime juice
2 tablespoons extra virgin olive oil, plus more for cooking
1 (1½–2-pound) flank steak

In a mortar, combine the salt, pepper, paprika, oregano, and garlic and smash the mixture with the pestle until it forms a paste. If you don't have a mortar and pestle, smash and chop the garlic very finely, then combine with the spices. Add the lime juice and olive oil and stir the marinade well.

Place the meat in a shallow dish and rub the marinade all over it. Cover and store in the fridge for at least 2 hours or as long as overnight. Take the meat out of the fridge about 30 minutes before cooking so that it can come to room temperature.

To a large cast-iron skillet, add just enough oil to cover the bottom of the pan. Let the pan sit over medium-high heat until the oil is smoking hot. While the pan is heating, wipe most of the marinade off of the steak and discard the marinade.

Carefully place the steak in the pan and cook it for 4 to 5 minutes on each side, until an instant-read thermometer inserted into the thickest part of the steak registers 130°F for medium rare. Transfer the steak to a cutting board and let it rest for 10 to 15 minutes.

Slice the steak into diagonal slices against the grain. Serve right away.

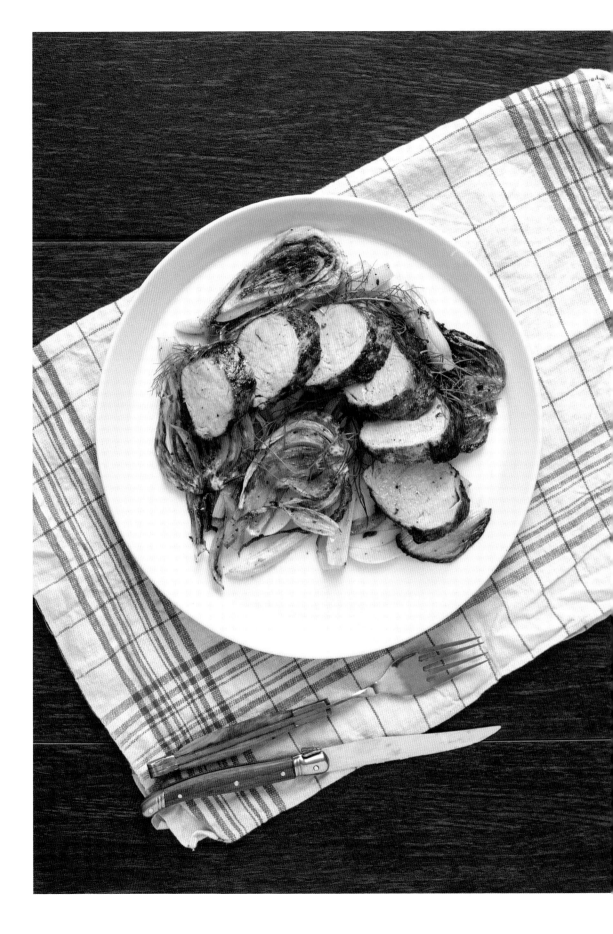

Pork Tenderloin with Caramelized Fennel

SERVES 6

Pork tenderloin is a wonderful lean and tender cut that is effectively fat-free, so it is a great way include pork in your diet without worrying. But, it can get a little boring. I had only ever eaten fennel raw, in salads, but then I saw a version of this recipe on the *Taste of Home* website, and it inspired me to try cooked fennel. Fennel turns out to be a wonderful pairing, and the roasting process enhances its natural sweetness.

¼ cup + 3 tablespoons extra virgin olive oil, divided
2 shallots, minced
3 teaspoons lemon zest
2 teaspoons kosher salt, divided
½ teaspoon red pepper flakes

1 teaspoon fresh thyme leaves
3 small pork tenderloins (2–3 pounds total)
3 medium bulbs fennel
½ teaspoon freshly ground black pepper
½ teaspoon granulated sugar

In a small bowl, mix together ¼ cup of the oil, the shallots, the lemon zest, 1 teaspoon of the salt, the red pepper flakes, and the thyme, blending well. Put the pork tenderloins into a gallon-size zip-top bag and add the marinade. Press out as much air as possible before sealing the bag, then smoosh the pork around in the bag until well coated. Transfer the bag to the fridge and let the pork marinate for at least 8 hours or as long as 24 hours.

Preheat the oven to 400°F. Line a baking sheet with aluminum foil and set aside.

Halve the fennel bulbs, discarding any damaged outer leaves. Remove the core and cut the fennel into ½-inch-thick slices. Transfer the fennel slices to a large bowl. Add 2 tablespoons of the olive oil, the remaining teaspoon of salt, the pepper, and the sugar, tossing until the fennel is completely coated.

Transfer the fennel to the prepared baking sheet and arrange it in a single layer, making sure that there is room around each fennel slice to avoid steaming. Roast, flipping the fennel slices once, for 30 to 35 minutes, until tender. Leave the fennel on the baking sheet.

Remove the tenderloins from the bag and discard the marinade. In a large nonstick skillet set over medium-high heat, heat the remaining tablespoon of oil until it shimmers. Add the pork and cook about 2 minutes per side, until browned. Place the browned pork on top of the roasted fennel, and return the baking sheet to the oven to roast for 18 to 22 minutes, until an instant-read thermometer inserted into the thickest part of the pork reads 145°F.

Let the pork rest at least 10 minutes before slicing. Serve slices on top of a portion of the caramelized fennel.

Turkey Cutlets with Mushrooms

SERVES 4

Healthy nutrition includes lots of lean protein. Turkey is a wonderful source of protein, but often it is relegated to holiday meals or deli counters. But, a healthy diet can incorporate turkey in many other ways. This quick dinner livens up turkey cutlets. You can also use the same recipe for veal or pork cutlets.

4 tablespoons all-purpose flour
½ teaspoon kosher salt, plus more to taste
¼ teaspoon freshly ground black pepper, plus more to taste
1½ pounds boneless, skinless turkey breast cutlets
4 tablespoons unsalted butter, divided
3 teaspoons grapeseed oil

2 tablespoons minced shallots
8 ounces cremini mushrooms, cleaned and sliced thin (see Note on page 145)
6 tablespoons dry white wine
2 tablespoons freshly squeezed lemon juice
2 tablespoons chopped fresh flat-leaf parsley
2 tablespoons toasted chopped walnuts (see Note on page 159), for garnish (optional)

Put the flour into a shallow baking dish and add the salt and pepper and mix well. Dredge the cutlets in the seasoned flour to get a thin coating, pat well to remove excess flour, and set aside in a single layer on a rack over a baking sheet. In a large nonstick skillet set over medium-high heat, melt 2 tablespoons of the butter and the grapeseed oil until the butter stops foaming. Add the turkey cutlets and cook on both sides, about 2 minutes per side, until golden brown. Transfer the cutlets to a plate.

Reduce the heat to medium-low. Add the shallots and sauté them in the remaining fat for about 2 minutes, until translucent and lightly browned. Add the mushrooms and sauté, stirring often, for 5 to 6 minutes, until they have released their juices, those juices have mostly evaporated, and the mushrooms have browned a bit.

Add the wine and lemon juice, stirring to combine, then add the remaining 2 tablespoons of butter, stirring gently but continuously to emulsify the butter into the sauce. Don't let the sauce sit still, or the butter will break and your sauce will be greasy.

When the butter is fully incorporated, slide the turkey cutlets back into the pan and cook for 2 to 3 minutes to finish heating through. Taste and add salt and pepper as needed.

Transfer the turkey cutlets to each of 4 plates, garnish with the mushroom sauce, parsley, and toasted walnuts, if using, and serve.

Chickpea Tagine with Sweet Potato

SERVES 8

Vegetarians often get short shrift, nutritionally. It can be hard for them to get enough protein in their diet, especially when they are eating at other people's homes, but this dish will solve that problem. A rich, comforting stew, this chickpea tagine is fantastically healthy and delicious enough to whip up for Meatless Monday. Serve over whole-wheat couscous or brown rice for a nutritionally complete meal.

⅓ cup canola oil
3 medium yellow onions, finely chopped
   (about 2 cups)
2 large sweet potatoes, peeled and cut into
   1½-inch chunks
4 medium cloves garlic, minced
1 tablespoon finely grated fresh ginger
1 teaspoon ground cumin
2 tablespoons tomato paste

1 teaspoon ground cinnamon
1–2 tablespoons harissa (see Note)
½ cup whole peeled almonds
½ cup dried apricots, coarsely chopped
3 (15-ounce) cans chickpeas, drained and
   rinsed
2½ cups homemade or store-bought low-
   sodium vegetable stock
1 teaspoon kosher salt, plus more to taste

In a large Dutch oven or heavy-bottomed stockpot set over medium-high heat, heat the oil until it shimmers. Add the onions and sweet potatoes and cook, stirring frequently, for 10 to 12 minutes, until the onions are golden and tender and the potatoes are beginning to brown at the edges. Transfer to a bowl and set aside.

Reduce the heat to medium. Add the garlic, ginger, cumin, tomato paste, cinnamon, and harissa. Sauté for about 1 minute, until the mixture changes from bright red to a deeper brick-like color. Add the almonds, apricots, and chickpeas and cook, stirring constantly, until the spicy paste coats everything.

Add the vegetable stock and salt. Bring the mixture to a boil and reduce the heat to medium-low. Simmer gently, stirring occasionally, for 12 to 15 minutes, until the potatoes are fork tender and the sauce has reduced and thickened slightly. Taste and add salt as needed.

Serve immediately.

NOTE: This can be a spicy dish, so start with 1 tablespoon of harissa, taste, and add more if your palate can handle it.

Whole-Wheat Orecchiette with Beans and Turkey Sausage

This hearty dish packs a double wallop of protein from beans and turkey sausage, and plenty of flavor! The whole-wheat pasta used here is both a flavorful and a healthful choice. The fiber is great for you, and the pasta's nuttiness and toothsome qualities stand up to the bold flavors in the dish.

1 pound whole-wheat orecchiette
4 tablespoons extra virgin olive oil, divided
1 pound Italian turkey sausage
1 (15-ounce) can cannellini beans, drained and rinsed
1 medium yellow onion, diced
Pinch red pepper flakes

4 cloves garlic, minced
½ teaspoon white wine vinegar
½ teaspoon freshly squeezed lemon juice
½ cup toasted walnuts (see Note on page 159)
Kosher salt and freshly ground black pepper, to taste
4 ounces ricotta salata, grated, for serving

Bring a large pot of salted water to a boil over medium-high heat. Add the pasta and cook for 8 to 10 minutes, until the pasta is al dente. Reserve 1 cup of the pasta water, drain the pasta, and set aside.

In a large sauté pan set over medium-high heat, heat 2 tablespoons of the oil until it shimmers. Add the sausage and sauté until it begins to lose its pinkness. Add the beans and continue to cook until the sausage starts to brown, about 3 minutes. Add the onion and red pepper flakes and sauté for 3 more minutes or until the onions are golden brown and the sausage is cooked through. Add the garlic and cook, stirring constantly, for 1 more minute and then remove the pan from the heat.

Add the vinegar and lemon juice, then the walnuts. Taste and add salt and pepper as needed. Because the sausage can be salty, you may not need much extra salt.

Add the drained pasta to the sausage mixture in the pan and toss to combine. Add the reserved pasta water, 2 tablespoons at a time, until everything comes together. You are looking for a very light sauce; the pasta should be barely glazed and not soupy.

Add the remaining 2 tablespoons of oil and toss to coat the pasta thoroughly. Transfer to a serving bowl. Top with the ricotta salata and serve hot.

Farro Salad with Pear, Blueberries, and Feta

SERVES 4 AS A SIDE

Farro is a nutty ancient grain that is great substitute for rice when you are in need of a change. Whole grains are the healthiest way to eat carbohydrates, since your body processes them slowly so they don't spike your blood sugar, and they provide excellent energy. This salad has a sweet-and-sour quality that makes it a great pairing for almost any meat.

1 cup farro (substitute wheat berries if you can't find farro)
1 tablespoon minced red onion
Freshly squeezed juice of 1 lemon
3 tablespoons white wine vinegar
2 tablespoons extra virgin olive oil

¼ cup chopped fresh basil
1 Bosc pear, peeled, cored, and diced
¾ cup crumbled feta
¼ cup dried blueberries
Kosher salt and freshly ground pepper, to taste

Bring a medium pot of salted water to a boil over high heat. Add the farro, reduce the heat to medium-low, and simmer the farro until it is al dente, about 20 minutes. Drain well and set aside.

While the farro cooks, in a small bowl combine the onion, lemon juice, and vinegar and let sit for 10 minutes. This will help temper some of the onion's bite. After it has soaked, add the olive oil and the basil and stir to combine, then set aside.

In a large bowl, toss together the farro, pear, feta, and blueberries until the salad is well mixed. Add the dressing and toss until everything is well coated. Taste and add salt and pepper as needed. Serve at room temperature.

Sautéed Mixed Greens

Dark, leafy greens are great for you and super diet friendly. With lots of vitamins and minerals, they are a superfood, and they are very low in calories, so you can eat a lot of them and know that you are doing something terrific for your body. Many dark, leafy greens are actually better for you when they are cooked and not raw, since the cooking helps your body break down the nutritional components. Now that you can buy prewashed bagged greens at your local grocery store, it is very easy to incorporate them into your diet. You can leave the fried shallots or onions off if you are extra concerned about fat, but as a garnish, they add great crunch and flavor.

1 pound fresh mixed greens, such as collard greens, mustard greens, and kale, washed and dried
2 tablespoons extra virgin olive oil
1 teaspoon vegetable oil

1 teaspoon red wine vinegar
Kosher salt and freshly ground pepper, to taste
½ cup fried shallots or onions, such as French's (optional)

Bring a large pot of salted water to a boil over medium-high heat. Stir in the greens and cook, uncovered, for 5 to 10 minutes.

Coarsely chop the greens.

In a large nonstick skillet set over medium-high heat, heat the olive oil and vegetable oil until they shimmer. Add the chopped greens and sauté until hot and wilted, about 4 minutes. Add the vinegar; taste and add salt and pepper as needed.

Transfer the greens to a bowl and garnish with the fried shallots, if using. Serve right away.

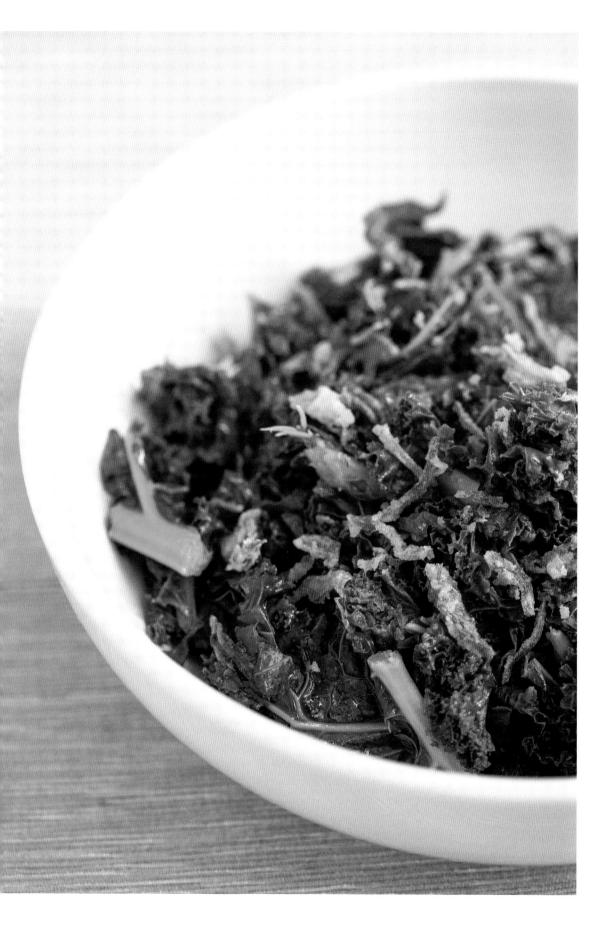

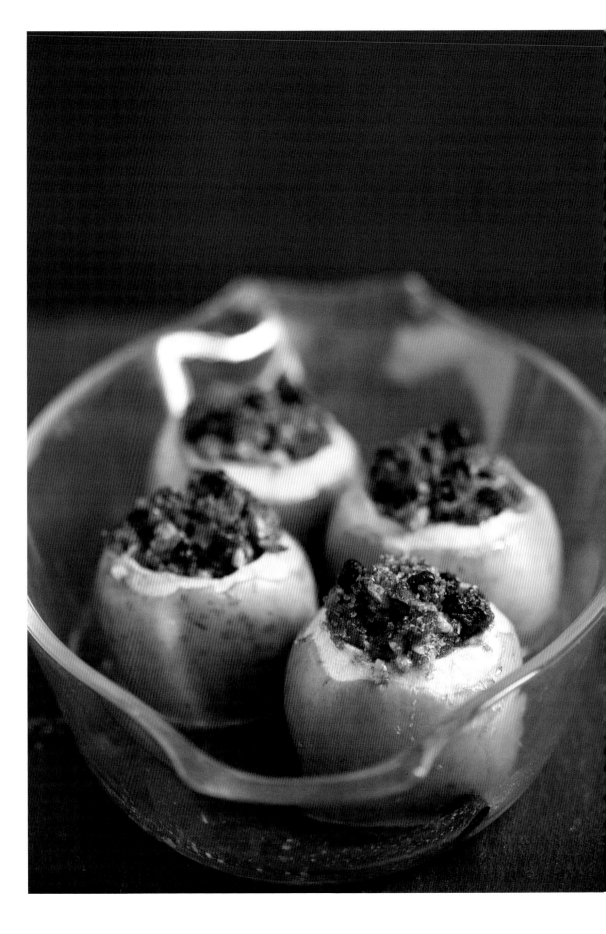

Baked Apples

Just because you are eating healthy doesn't mean you don't want or deserve dessert! In fact, they say that people who continue to plan for treats like this in their diet are more likely to stay with their program, because they don't feel deprived. But desserts can be difficult; often baked goods are full of sugar and refined grains. These baked apples are a guiltless treat—and perfectly preportioned. If you are serving people who aren't watching their diets as closely, you can add a scoop of vanilla or cinnamon ice cream, or a dollop of whipped cream or crème fraîche. This is the perfect dessert for a dinner party, but it also makes a healthy breakfast when paired with vanilla Greek yogurt.

⅓ cup firmly packed brown sugar
1 teaspoon ground cinnamon
¼ teaspoon kosher salt
½ cup toasted chopped walnuts (see Note
   on page 159)

½ cup raisins
6 good-quality firm apples, such as Fuji
¾ cup apple cider

Preheat the oven to 400°F.

In a small bowl, mix together the sugar, cinnamon, and salt until well combined. Add the walnuts and raisins and toss until the nuts and fruit are well coated. Set the filling aside.

Using a melon baller or a grapefruit spoon, remove the cores from the apples without cutting through the bottom; leave about a ½ inch of the flesh intact at the bottom of the apple to contain the filling. Scoop out just enough flesh to leave a solid wall of apple all the way around.

Put an equal amount of the filling into each of the apples and arrange them in an oval au gratin dish or a 9 × 13-inch baking dish so that each apple has space around it. This will help the apples cook evenly.

Add the apple cider to the bottom of the dish; it should come about ½ inch up the sides of the apples. Cover the dish with aluminum foil and bake for 10 minutes. Remove the foil and continue to bake, uncovered, for another 20 to 25 minutes, until the apples are tender but still holding their shape and the juices have reduced a bit.

Remove the dish from the oven. Let the apples cool in the dish for at least 15 minutes. Serve warm in shallow bowls with the juices spooned over the tops.

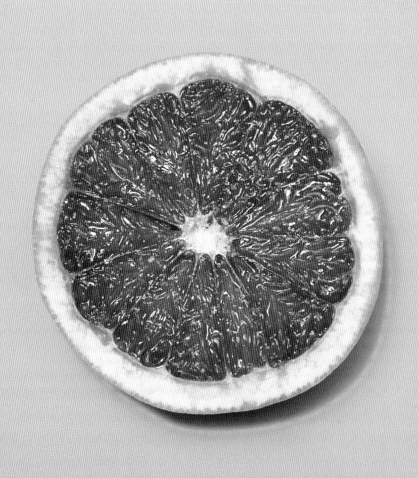

CHAPTER 7: Protectoral Wellness

PROTECTORAL WELLNESS IS ABOUT **SAFEGUARDING**. It means being authentically aware of hazards at home, work, school, and within your community. Doing so is empowering, and if you truly pay attention, you can prevent the onset of accidents, injuries, and illnesses. It is not enough to simply remind yourself to pay closer attention to your surroundings. Instead, you should consider actually practicing awareness. In your home, this can be accomplished by identifying one thing each day that you never took notice of before—a chip of paint or blemish on a wall, the uneven wear in a carpeted room, a unique smell in the kitchen, or literally anything else you've never noticed before. In other words, if you do the reps in the gym to get physically stronger, then doing your awareness reps makes you protectorally well!

COOKING for your protectoral well-being (and with all cooking, for that matter) means safeguarding everything you use when preparing food. It also means being aware of the safety of everyone else within your sphere of food prep. Several important considerations come to mind. These include keeping your hot ingredients hot and your cold ones cold until they are actually used in order to prevent the growth of harmful bacteria. Never thaw frozen foods at room temperature; do so in the fridge, even though it takes longer. Additionally, wash (don't rinse) counters, cutting boards, utensils, and your hands before and after food prep. When working with raw meats, poultry, seafood, or eggs, be sure to either use different utensils and equipment or to thoroughly wash every item (including your hands!) that came into contact with the raw item to prevent cross-contamination. Keep an eye and a nose on the ingredients in your fridge and cabinets, and most important, if you have a moment where you believe something either smells or tastes off, even just a little bit, chuck it and make a new decision—even if that decision is that it's Pizza Night! Trust me, 90 percent of foodborne illness can be prevented by just being smart and careful in your kitchen. Finally, be aware of any food allergies and/or intolerances that you and or your eating companions may have.

EATING for your protectoral well-being means eating foods that boost your immune system and otherwise help keep you and your loved ones safe and healthy. The recipes within this chapter contain foods proven to have health and medical benefits. Some (green leafy veggies, fresh fruits) are loaded with antioxidants while others (salmon, olive oil) contain essential fatty acids. I also chose ingredients that are packed with vitamins and other nutrients that, when consumed as whole foods (as opposed to supplements), have extraordinary medicinal benefits.

Ninety percent of foodborne illness can be prevented by just being smart and careful in your kitchen.

Stuffed Mushrooms

SERVES 6

Button mushrooms are often pooh-poohed for being boring, from a culinary perspective; however, they are great for boosting your immune system, as they are chock-full of antioxidants, B vitamins, and most importantly, selenium. A selenium deficiency has been linked to an increased susceptibility to severe flus. I first started making a version of this recipe when I read it in *Real Simple*. However, many stuffed mushroom recipes, including that one, rely on cheese or buttery béchamel sauce to bind the filling. In order to make this recipe more healthful, I have adapted it to use hummus as the binder, which also adds protein and creaminess. These mushrooms are a fast and easy appetizer, great for parties during the cold and flu season!

18 medium button mushrooms, cleaned (see Note on page 145)
2 tablespoons extra virgin olive oil, plus more for drizzling
2 cloves garlic, finely minced
½ red onion, finely minced

1 (10-ounce) package frozen chopped spinach, thawed and squeezed dry
½ cup plain hummus
1 teaspoon lemon zest
Kosher salt and finely ground black pepper, to taste
1 cup breadcrumbs, divided

Preheat the oven to 400°F. Line a large baking sheet with aluminum foil, spray it with nonstick spray, and set it aside.

Remove and reserve all of the mushroom stems by holding the cap in one hand and gently twisting the stem with the other until the cap pops off. Using a small spoon, scrape the gills (reserving them for the next step) from the underside of the mushrooms until you have created a nice cup for the filling.

Mince the stems and gills together, transfer to a bowl, and set aside. Arrange the mushroom caps, cavity-side down, on the prepared baking sheet and spray the tops lightly with nonstick spray. Roast for 8 to 10 minutes, until the mushrooms are lightly browned and just tender, but not too soft. Remove them from the oven and set them aside.

In a medium nonstick skillet set over medium heat, heat the oil until it shimmers. Add the garlic, onion, and chopped mushroom stems and gills. Sauté, stirring constantly, for 4 to 5 minutes, until the onion is lightly golden brown and the mushroom bits have released and mostly cooked off their juices. Add the spinach and cook until heated through and the rest of the moisture has evaporated.

Transfer the spinach mixture to a medium bowl. Stir in the hummus and the lemon zest. Taste the filling and add salt and pepper as needed. Add ½ cup of the breadcrumbs, stirring until well mixed.

Flip the mushroom caps so that the cup side is facing up. Using a pair of spoons or a small cookie scoop, fill each mushroom cap with the spinach filling, 1 to 2 tablespoons depending on the size of your mushrooms. They can mound up a bit. Sprinkle the remaining ½ cup breadcrumbs on top of the stuffed mushrooms. Drizzle a few drops of the olive oil on top of the breadcrumbs, and transfer the baking sheet back into the oven. Bake for 10 to 13 minutes, until golden brown.

Serve the stuffed mushrooms hot or at room temperature.

Spicy Chicken–Garlic Soup

Chicken soup is called "Jewish penicillin" for a reason: it has natural anti-inflammatory properties and a host of other health benefits, in addition to being soothing. I've added an immunity boost by increasing the amount of garlic and adding dark, leafy greens and chiles. Spicy foods are good when you have a cold, as they help drain your sinuses and appeal to a palate that is dulled by illness. This recipe makes a large batch because this soup freezes beautifully, so you can eat half and save half for the next time you feel a cold coming on!

2 heads garlic, cloves separated and peeled (see Note on page 181)

1 pound mustard greens, collard greens, kale, or spinach leaves

4 tablespoons extra virgin olive oil

2 medium yellow onions, diced

2 small red Thai chiles, seeded and finely minced

4 ribs celery, diced

4 carrots, peeled and diced

2 tablespoons lemon zest

3 quarts homemade or store-bought low-sodium chicken stock

Kosher salt and freshly ground black pepper, to taste

Pinch red pepper flakes (optional)

2 tablespoons chopped fresh flat-leaf parsley

2 cups diced cooked chicken

2 cups cooked orzo pasta or brown rice

Slice the garlic cloves as thinly as you can and set aside. Wash the greens and, while still a little wet, put them in a medium high-sided skillet. Set the skillet over medium-high heat and cover. When you see steam leaking around the lid, remove it and stir the greens down. Continue to cook, uncovered, until the leaves are wilted. Drain any excess liquid using a strainer, and chop the greens roughly. You should have about 2 cups.

In a Dutch oven set over medium-low heat, heat the oil until it shimmers. Add the onions and cook until they are just translucent. Add the garlic and chiles and stir. Be careful not to have your face over the pan when you add the chiles; the spicy fumes can irritate to your eyes and nose.

Add the celery, carrots, and lemon zest and sauté for about 5 minutes. Add the stock and chopped cooked greens. Increase the heat to high and bring the mixture to a boil. Reduce the heat to medium-high and cook, stirring occasionally, for about 20 minutes, until the vegetables are cooked through and the broth is fragrant. Taste the soup and add salt and pepper as needed. Add the red pepper flakes, if using, to increase the spice level.

Stir in the cooked chicken and orzo and cook just long enough to heat through. Serve hot. Leftovers will keep up to 5 days in the fridge in an airtight container, or in the freezer for up to 2 months.

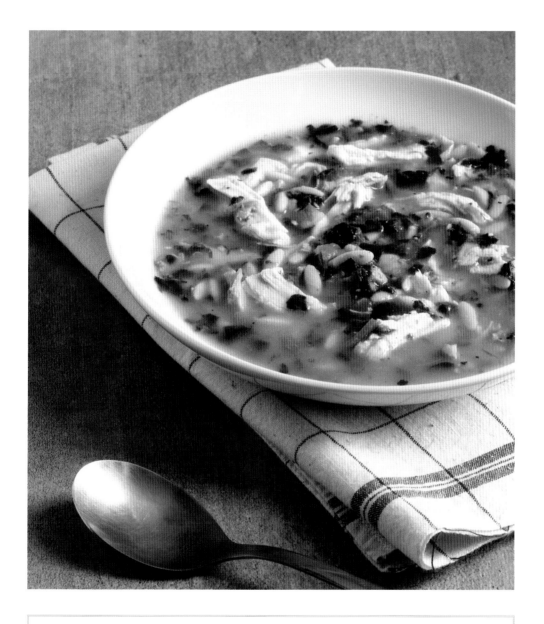

NOTE: When peeling this many garlic cloves, I use an old chef's trick. Get a pair of large (this is important) metal bowls—they should be the same size or as close to it as you can get. Break apart the heads of garlic and put all of the cloves into one bowl. Turn the other metal bowl over on top to make sort of a sphere. Using your hands to keep the two bowls tightly together, shake the garlic cloves as hard and fast as you can for about a minute. When you stop, you should find that the cloves have all separated from their skins like magic! Run cold water into the bowl, so that the skins float up and you can easily remove them. Then drain the cloves, pat them dry with paper towels, and continue with the recipe.

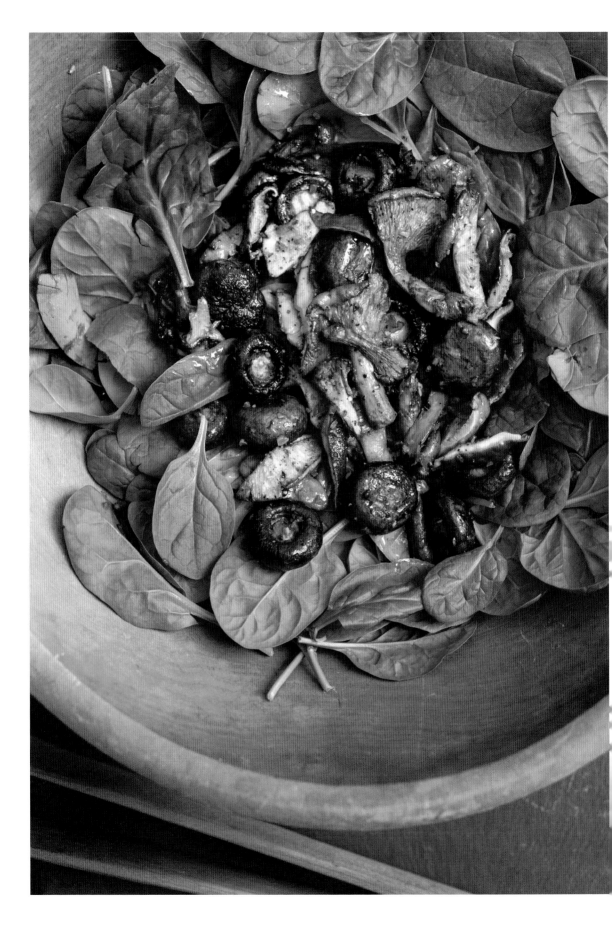

Spinach Salad with Roasted Mushrooms

Spinach and mushrooms are more than just a great flavor combination; they are a one-two punch of vitamins and minerals like vitamin A, vitamin D, vitamin E, potassium, magnesium, folate, iron, and zinc. This salad is a great lunch or starter for a dinner.

⅓ pound button mushrooms, cleaned and chopped (see Note on page 145)

⅓ pound cremini mushrooms, cleaned and chopped

⅓ pound chanterelle mushrooms, cleaned and chopped

¼ cup peanut oil

3 shallots, minced

2 tablespoons unsalted butter, melted

Kosher salt and freshly ground black pepper, to taste

¼ cup extra virgin olive oil

¼ cup red or white wine vinegar

1 tablespoon Dijon mustard

1 pound fresh baby spinach leaves, washed well and dried

Preheat the oven to 350°F. Line a large roasting pan with aluminum foil and set aside.

In a medium bowl, combine all the mushrooms with the peanut oil, tossing to coat. Transfer to the prepared roasting pan. Sprinkle the shallots over the mushroom mixture and then drizzle the butter over everything. Season well with salt and pepper. Roast the mushrooms for 30 to 40 minutes, until they are browned and fragrant.

Meanwhile, in a small bowl, mix together the olive oil, vinegar, and mustard until well combined. While the mushrooms are still hot, add the vinaigrette and stir to combine.

Serve warm on a bed of the baby spinach, with any extra juices spooned over.

Chicken in Vinegar

SERVES 4

Your gastrointestinal tract is a big part of your body's immune system. You want the friendly bacteria in your gut to flourish, as it helps your gut work efficiently and protect your health. The type of acid found in apple cider vinegar has antiviral properties. I have always just used vinegar in salad dressings, but when I saw a version of this recipe in *Saveur* magazine, I wondered if it might be a good way to incorporate it into my diet in different ways. The traditional recipe calls for red wine vinegar, which doesn't have the health benefits of apple cider vinegar. Cooking chicken with apple cider vinegar is a terrific way of incorporating this healthy ingredient into your diet. If you aren't as concerned about the immune-system benefits, you can swap it out for sherry vinegar or the traditional red wine vinegar for a different flavor profile.

2 pounds bone-in, skin-on chicken thighs
Kosher salt and freshly ground black pepper, to taste
3 tablespoons clarified butter or ghee
1 tablespoon grapeseed oil
4 medium shallots, minced
⅓ cup + 1 tablespoon organic apple cider vinegar, divided
⅔ cup dry hard cider, preferably French
1 tablespoon dark agave syrup

¾ cup homemade or store-bought low-sodium chicken stock
1 tablespoon tomato paste
¼ teaspoon ground nutmeg
½ teaspoon sweet paprika
1 tablespoon fresh thyme leaves
2 tablespoons unsalted butter, cold, cut into cubes
1 tablespoon chopped fresh flat-leaf parsley

Season the chicken on all sides with salt and pepper. In a large frying pan set over medium-high heat, heat the ghee until it shimmers. In batches, add the chicken and cook until golden brown on both sides, 3 to 4 minutes per side. Transfer the chicken to a plate and set aside. Reserve the ghee and chicken fat from the pan in a small bowl. When the fat has solidified you can discard it or save to use for cooking potatoes.

Return the pan to medium-high heat, add the grapeseed oil, and heat until it shimmers. Add the shallots and sauté for 3 to 4 minutes, until they are tender. Pour ⅓ cup of the vinegar, the cider, and the agave syrup into the pan. Increase the heat to high and bring the mixture to a boil. Reduce the heat to medium. Keeping an eye on it and stirring frequently, reduce the liquid by about one-third.

Meanwhile, in a small bowl, whisk together the stock, tomato paste, nutmeg, paprika, and thyme.

When the vinegar mixiture has reduced, add the stock mixture, increase the heat to medium-high, and bring it back to a boil. Reduce the heat to medium-low. Add the chicken pieces back to the pan, nestling them into the sauce. Increase the heat to medium-high and bring the mixture back to a boil, then cover the pan and reduce the heat to low. Braise the chicken for 35 to 40 minutes, until the chicken is tender but not falling apart.

Transfer the chicken from the sauce to a warm serving platter. Increase the heat to high and reduce the sauce, stirring constantly, for 4 to 5 minutes, until it is thick and shiny. Reduce the heat to medium. Add the cold butter, a couple of cubes at a time, whisking constantly so that the butter emulsifies into the sauce and doesn't just melt and make it greasy. As soon as all of the butter is fully incorporated, remove the pan from the heat. Stir in the remaining tablespoon of vinegar. Taste the sauce and add salt and pepper as needed.

Pour the sauce over the chicken on the platter and garnish with the parsley. Serve hot.

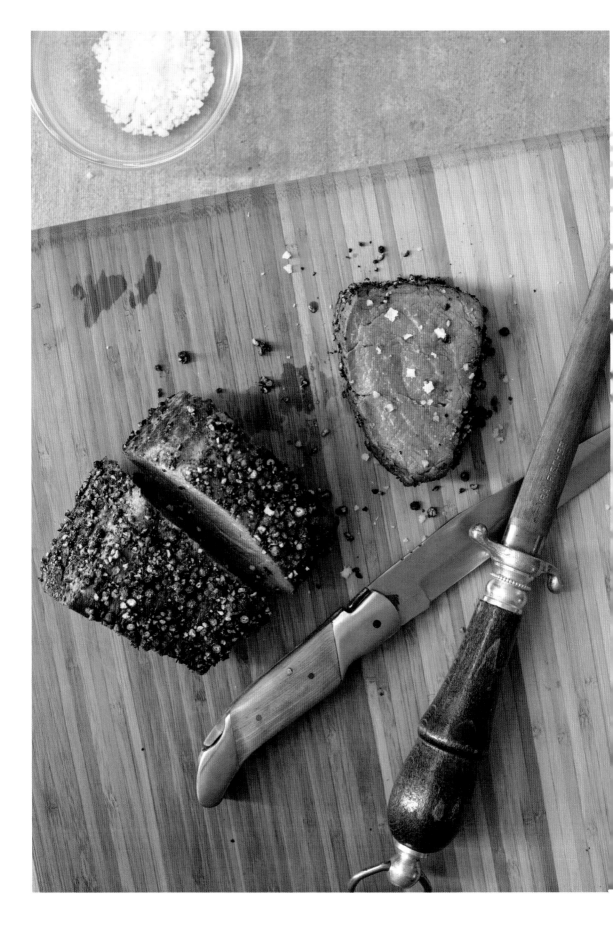

Peppercorn-Crusted Filet

SERVES 6

Black peppercorns are good for immunity. They stimulate the signaling molecule that primes the body to fight off viruses and they support the function of our white blood cells, enhancing their ability to create antibodies. The white blood cells are the majority of our immune system, which means that keeping them functioning at their highest levels has the potential to have a cancer-preventing effect. However, it's usually difficult to incorporate a generous amount of peppercorns into a dish. *America's Test Kitchen*, famous for its commitment to finding the best way to cook everything, figured out how to create black peppercorn crusts that avoid the mouth-numbing effects of raw peppercorns and their tendency to burn when patted onto the outside of meat. In this recipe, I have adapted their technique of cooking the peppercorns first in oil, which infuses the oil and tempers the peppercorns' heat. This technique can be used with other proteins as well.

6 tablespoons black peppercorns
6 tablespoons + 2 teaspoons extra virgin olive
    oil, divided

1½ tablespoons kosher salt
1 (48-ounce) center-cut filet mignon roast
Flaky sea salt, such as Maldon, for garnish

Using a mortar and pestle, lightly crush the peppercorns to form a coarse mixture, with some peppercorns merely cracked in half and some in smaller pieces. Don't crush too much or you will end up with too fine a mixture. Transfer the peppercorn pieces to a small strainer and shake to just filter out the smallest powdery bits.

In a small saucepan set over low heat, heat 4 tablespoons of the oil until it shimmers. Add the crushed peppercorns and cook for 5 to 6 minutes, until they begin to smell nutty. Transfer the peppercorns and oil to a small bowl and let cool to room temperature. Then stir in the kosher salt and set aside.

Place a large sheet of plastic wrap, about 3 inches longer than the roast, on a work surface. Spread the peppercorn–oil mixture onto the plastic, in the shape of a rectangle larger than the roast. Place the roast in the center of the plastic wrap and pull its sides up and over the roast, creating an even coating. Close up the plastic and roll the roast firmly back and forth on the work surface to press the mixture into the roast. Twist the ends of the plastic wrap tightly and store in the fridge for 15 minutes.

Preheat the oven to 450°F.

CONTINUED ▷

Peppercorn-Crusted Filet

CONTINUED

In a heavy-bottomed nonstick skillet set over medium-high heat, heat the remaining 2 tablespoons plus 2 teaspoons oil until it shimmers. Remove the roast carefully from the plastic wrap; it should have a good coating of the peppercorn mixture, but don't worry if some falls off. Add the roast to the skillet and cook for 3 to 4 minutes per side, turning gently so as to not disturb the coating too much, until browned on all sides.

Transfer the pan to the oven and roast for an additional 10 minutes, until an instant-read thermometer inserted into the thickest part of the roast registers 125°F for medium rare.

Transfer the roast to a wire rack and let it rest for at least 12 to 15 minutes. Slice into 6 equal steaks. Garnish with a sprinkle of sea salt.

Oysters with Pomegranate Mignonette

Oysters might be famous for their impact on your libido, but they are also wonderful for supporting your immune system. Oysters are full of zinc; you know, that stuff you take to ward off the common cold or lessen its duration? This is a much more pleasurable way to get your zinc on. A mignonette is a classic French vinaigrette that is specifically designed for oysters and really enhances their briny flavor.

4 dozen fresh oysters, scrubbed
¾ cup champagne vinegar
4 tablespoons pomegranate juice
2 small shallots, very finely minced

1 teaspoon granulated sugar
½ cup pomegranate seeds (see Note on page 15), for garnish

To shuck the oysters, hold them tight to the counter with a towel in your hand. Using a shucking knife, pop the hinge of the shell and then run the knife along the inside of the top shell to release the oyster. (If you have never done this before, you might want to enlist a friend who has, or look up a video online to see how it is done.) Set the oysters, in their shells, on a platter of crushed ice.

In a small bowl, whisk together the vinegar, pomegranate juice, shallots, and sugar. Cover and let sit for up to 3 hours at room temperature, or store in the fridge for up to 24 hours.

Arrange 12 oysters on each of 4 plates. Pour a small spoonful of the sauce over each oyster. Garnish with 2 to 3 pomegranate seeds per oyster and serve.

Sweet and Sour Cabbage Rolls

SERVES 4 FOR DINNER OR 8 AS AN APPETIZER

Cabbage has wonderful healthy properties, including being a good source of vitamins B1 and B2, which help support your immune system. It is also a good source of dietary fiber, which will help keep your digestive system working smoothly. But there are more interesting ways to get cabbage into your diet besides slaw. Here, it serves as a wrap for a flavorful sweet-and-sour turkey dish. Be sure to buy ground turkey thighs—not ground turkey breast—as you need the dark meat for its moisture.

1 head savoy cabbage
3 quarts water
2 tablespoons extra virgin olive oil
1 medium yellow onion, chopped small
1 carrot, peeled and grated
1 rib celery, thinly sliced
1 parsnip, peeled and grated

Kosher salt and freshly ground black pepper, to taste
1 pound ground turkey thigh
½ cup long grain white rice
2 tablespoons tomato paste
4 cups tomato sauce, tomato juice, or V8
3 tablespoons dark brown sugar
2 teaspoons red wine vinegar

Using a small paring knife, core the cabbage from the bottom, but leave the head whole. Place the cabbage upside-down in a large heatproof bowl. In a large pot, bring the water to a boil over high heat. Pour the water over the cabbage and let it sit for 10 minutes. Drain the cabbage and set it aside. This will soften the cabbage just enough to allow you to easily wrap your rolls, since raw cabbage would snap and tear.

In a large high-sided sauté pan set over medium-high heat, heat the oil until it shimmers. Add the onion and cook for about 5 minutes, until it is soft and lightly golden brown. Add the carrot, celery, and parsnip and sauté them for about 2 minutes, until they are soft. Taste and add salt and pepper as needed, then transfer the mixture to a bowl and let it cool a bit. Add the turkey, rice, and tomato paste and mix to combine. Season again with salt and pepper.

Pull off the large outer leaves of the cabbage and cut out the large center stalk so that each leaf can be rolled easily. If the leaf is very large, halve it to make 2 rolls; if it is smaller, partially cut out the stalk and pull the sides to overlap before you roll it up. Pat the leaves dry with paper towels.

Place ¼ to ⅓ cup of the filling in each leaf. Roll the leaf up by tucking the bottom of it over the top of the filling, then folding in the 2 sides and rolling tightly up until the filling is completely enclosed. Arrange the rolls, seam-side down, in the same sauté pan you cooked the vegetables in. In a separate small bowl, mix together the tomato sauce, sugar, and vinegar. Add just enough of this mixture to the pan to cover the rolls; you may not need all of the mixture.

Bring to a boil over medium-high heat. Reduce the heat to low, cover, and let the rolls simmer for about 45 minutes.

Serve immediately. If the sauce needs thinning, you can add a bit of water, or any juice you didn't use, and then pour the sauce over the rolls before you serve.

Immunity Smoothie

SERVES 1

These days a lot of attention is being given to the health benefits of "green" smoothies. I'm not saying that there isn't a health benefit to them, but I've yet to meet one that is truly crave worthy. For me, satiety is primary in all things, and if you are going to substitute a smoothie for an actual meal, I think it should be yummy. This smoothie is full of immunity-boosting ingredients—such as yogurt, blueberries, dark chocolate, honey, and cinnamon—but mostly it tastes great and will fill you up and energize you. You might be curious about why I use dairy milk here, as many people think that dairy is bad for you. However, the calcium in cow's milk can help your immune system, since it allows you to better process vitamin D, which is wonderful for your system. Many commercial nut milks, while promoted as good substitutes, contain 2 percent or less of the nuts in question, which means that you don't actually get the same health benefits as you would by just eating the nut.

1 cup 2% milk, plus more as needed
½ cup full-fat plain Greek yogurt
½ cup fresh or frozen blueberries, plus more as needed
1 tablespoon dark cocoa powder

¼ teaspoon ground cinnamon
2 drops pure vanilla extract
½ ripe banana, cut into chunks and frozen, plus more as needed
1 teaspoon honey

Put all of the ingredients into your blender and purée until smooth. If it's too thick, add more milk; if it's too thin, add more blueberries or banana. Serve right away.

Savory Vegetable Crumble with Oats

SERVES 6

Most people think of fruit desserts when they hear the word *crumble*—I know I did—but then I saw a version of this recipe by noted food photographer Matt Armendariz, and it opened my mind to the savory side of crumbles! The combination of healthy veggies with an oat-crumble topping makes for a hearty and fiber-packed vegetarian main dish that will help boost your immune system while satisfying your hunger!

Filling

6 cups mixed cooked vegetables, coarsely
   chopped
2 cups canned white beans, drained and rinsed
4 plum tomatoes, roughly chopped
1 medium yellow onion, chopped
1 clove garlic, minced
2 tablespoons extra virgin olive oil
1 teaspoon kosher salt
½ teaspoon freshly ground black pepper

Crumble Topping

½ cup all-purpose flour
¼ cup whole-wheat flour
½ teaspoon kosher salt
¼ teaspoon freshly ground black pepper
½ teaspoon mustard powder
1 teaspoon chopped fresh rosemary
6 tablespoons unsalted butter, cold, cut into
   ½-inch cubes
¾ cup toasted rolled oats (see Note on page 159)
½ cup grated Cheddar
3 teaspoons buttermilk, cold

Preheat the oven to 400°F. Spray a 9 × 13-inch baking dish with nonstick spray and set it aside.

To make the filling, put the mixed vegetables in a large bowl. Stir in the beans, tomatoes, onion, and garlic. Drizzle the olive oil over the mixture and add the salt and pepper. Stir the mixture until everything is well combined and set it aside.

To make the crumble topping, put the all-purpose flour, whole-wheat flour, salt, pepper, mustard powder, and rosemary in the bowl of a food processor. Pulse twice to combine. Sprinkle the cold butter cubes around in the bowl. Pulse until you get a crumbly texture, about 8 more pulses. Transfer the mixture to a large bowl and add the oats and cheese, stirring together the mixture with a fork so that it does not clump. Pour the buttermilk over the mixture, using the fork to just stir it through. You should have some small crumbles and some sandy texture; it should be very loose and not like a batter.

Pour the vegetable filling into the prepared baking dish, spreading it evenly over the bottom. Spoon the crumble topping over the vegetables in an even layer. Transfer to the oven and cook, uncovered, for 40 minutes, or until the vegetables are soft and the topping is crispy and browned. Start checking it at about 30 minutes just to be safe.

Let rest for 10 minutes before serving hot.

Carrots with Walnuts and Cinnamon

SERVES 4 AS A SIDE

Carrots are a great source of beta-carotene, walnuts are full of antioxidants, and cinnamon is antiviral, antifungal, and antibacterial. Together, they are simply delicious.

1 pound carrots, peeled
2 tablespoons extra virgin olive oil
1 tablespoon ground cinnamon

Kosher salt and freshly ground black pepper, to taste
½ cup toasted chopped walnuts (see Note on page 159)

Preheat the oven to 400°F. Toss the carrots with the olive oil. Arrange them in a single layer on a baking sheet. Sprinkle them with the cinnamon and season with salt and pepper. Roast for 35 to 45 minutes, until the carrots are tender and golden brown.

Transfer the carrots to a serving platter, sprinkle them with the walnuts, and serve warm.

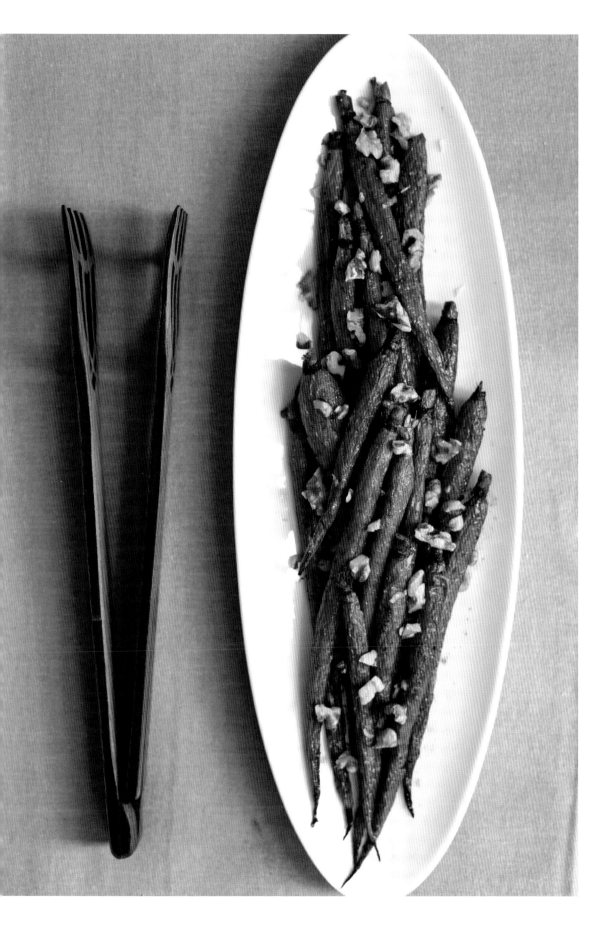

Herbed Barley with Lemon

Barley is loaded with beta-glucan, a special fiber compound that has powerful antioxidant properties. Consuming barley can help the body resist the flu, speed up healing time if you have an injury, and boost the immune system. Fiber helps keep your digestive system running smoothly. This simple side dish pairs well with any protein and is a nice break from typical rice or potatoes.

1 tablespoon vegetable oil
1 medium onion, chopped
1¼ cups homemade or store-bought low-sodium chicken or beef stock
¾ cup water
1 cup pearl barley

1 tablespoon lemon zest
½ teaspoon dried thyme
Kosher salt and freshly ground black pepper, to taste
1 tablespoon chopped fresh flat-leaf parsley
1 tablespoon chopped chives

In a large saucepan set over medium-high heat, heat the oil until it shimmers. Add the onion and sauté until tender, about 3 minutes.

Add the stock, water, barley, lemon zest, and thyme and stir to combine. Bring the mixture to a boil. Reduce the heat to low, cover, and simmer for about 25 minutes, or until the liquid has been almost completely absorbed and the barley is tender.

Taste and add salt and pepper as needed. Transfer to a serving dish, toss with the parsley and chives, and serve warm.

Ginger Sweet Potatoes

Sweet potatoes are a great immunity-boosting food, as are ginger and cinnamon since they naturally help the body rid itself of toxins. This sweet and savory side dish pairs well with poultry and pork.

⅔ cup homemade or store-bought low-sodium chicken stock
½ teaspoon ground cinnamon
½ tablespoon pure maple syrup
½ tablespoon soy sauce
1 tablespoon ginger jam (see Note)
1 tablespoon extra virgin olive oil

1 medium yellow onion, chopped
2 tablespoons finely minced fresh ginger
4 medium sweet potatoes, peeled and cut into 1-inch chunks
Kosher salt and freshly ground black pepper, to taste

In a small bowl, mix together the stock, cinnamon, maple syrup, soy sauce, and ginger jam until well blended.

In a large Dutch oven set over medium-high heat, heat the oil until it shimmers. Add the onion and sauté for about 3 minutes, until it is translucent. Add the ginger and continue to cook, stirring constantly, until the mixture is fragrant and beginning to brown.

Add the sweet potatoes to the Dutch oven and stir to combine well. Pour in the stock mixture and stir well. Bring the mixture to a boil. Reduce the heat to low and simmer, covered, for 15 to 20 minutes, until the potatoes are tender all the way through but not mushy.

Remove the lid and continue to cook, stirring occasionally, for 3 to 4 minutes, until the liquid reduces to a glaze over the potatoes. Taste and add salt and pepper as needed, then transfer to a large serving bowl and serve hot.

> **NOTE:** If you can't find ginger jam, use apricot jam mixed with 1 teaspoon ground ginger as a substitute.

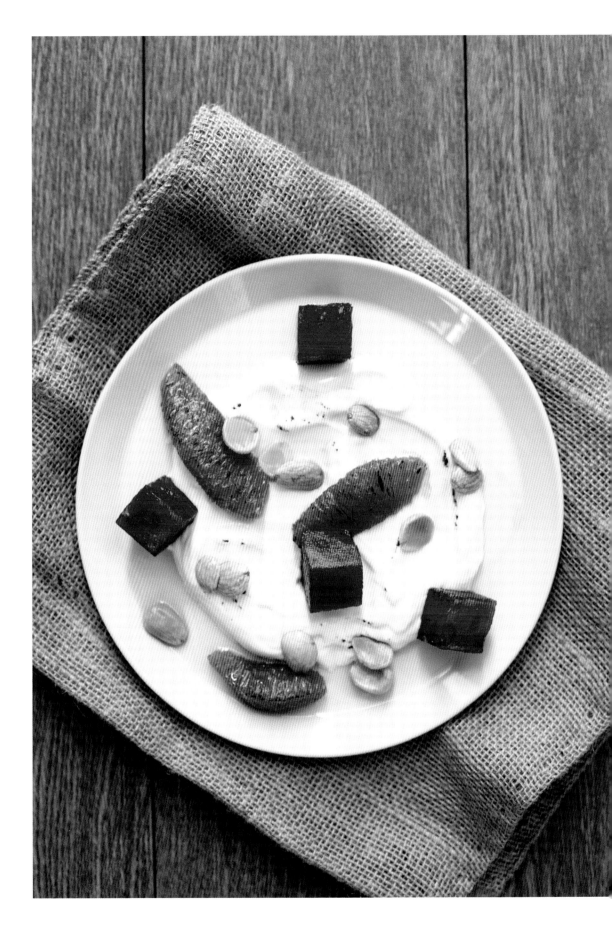

Skyr with Almonds and Honey-Brûléed Grapefruit and Watermelon

SERVES 4

Skyr is an Icelandic style of yogurt that is a terrific source of probiotics, protein, and calcium. Many doctors believe that a healthy gut with good flora is key to overall health, but especially for preventing colds and flu. Almonds are full of vitamin E, and watermelon and grapefruit have magnesium, antioxidants, and vitamin C. They also taste great together! This simple summer dessert is low in calories, high in health benefits, and completely refreshing.

12 ounces vanilla-flavored skyr, like Siggi's
1 small red grapefruit, supremed (see Lemon–
   Caper Salsa on page 160)

1 cup cubed watermelon
4 teaspoons honey
4 tablespoons chopped Marcona almonds

Spread about 3 ounces of the skyr, or a heaping ¼ cup, on each of 4 medium plates. Arrange about 4 of the grapefruit segments and 3 to 4 of the watermelon cubes on each plate. Using a spoon or clean finger, drizzle a thin coating of honey (about 1 teaspoon) over the tops of the grapefruit and watermelon.

Using a small kitchen torch, scorch the honey so that it gets browned and creates a crackly crust on the fruit.

Sprinkle 1 tablespoon of the chopped almonds onto each plate and serve immediately.

> **NOTE:** Instead of using a whole grapefruit, you can use store-bought red grapefruit segments packed in juice—just be sure to drain them well and pat dry.

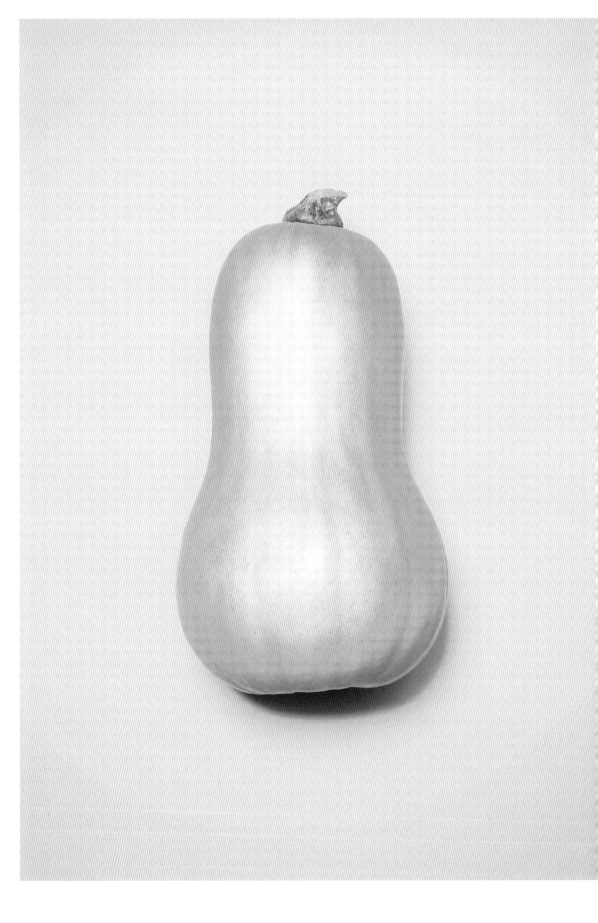

CHAPTER 8: Social Wellness

SOCIAL WELLNESS IS ABOUT **RELATING**. It is about attracting and maintaining quality, long-lasting relationships. We all know the importance of this for our well-being about as much as we realize how challenging it can be. The essentials to any quality relationship include love (affection), communication (exchange), trust (confidence), and intimacy (closeness). Consider each of these a continuum of sorts. For example, you need only a small amount of these four relational ingredients for acquaintances but a higher amount for your family and your significant other. Cooking at home can truly be the key to enriching all four of these—and to ultimately nurturing your social well-being.

COOKING for your social well-being means cooking for social gatherings and cooking with other people as a way of connecting. It can be the perfect way to spend quality time with those important to you and give them the attention that they deserve. Use the four ingredients to quality relationships as a way to infuse social wellness into the cooking process. Add some *love* to the occasion by sending out an affectionate invitation to an intimate cooking experience. Greet the person with a warm embrace before you begin. Make the cooking process *communicative* by sharing thoughts and ideas along the way—be it suggestions for swapping out an ingredient, or talking about other people in your lives who might love the dish—and, just maybe, share a secret or two! Many recipes in this chapter lend themselves to being constructed by two people. When doing so, remember to *trust* your cooking partner, even when you question his or her methods. It can be a good exercise for those of you who might be working on issues of control to give yourself over to being the sous chef or second in command and let your cooking partner take the lead. Finally, remain appropriately *intimate* during the cooking process. You are choosing to connect, and whether it is working with your grandmother to learn a secret family recipe, making cookies with your kids for the school bake sale, or creating a romantic evening with your partner full of playful tastes, intimacy is supported and encouraged. So take this opportunity to shut off the television, put your phones aside, and talk. Too many people these days are so "connected" to their screens that they forget to actually connect in real life.

EATING for your social well-being is about enjoying foods that lend themselves to being shared. This means that during mealtime, romantic dinners for two, dinner parties with friends, and large family-style feasts all provide the perfect opportunity to enhance the social experience. The tasty recipes in this chapter lend themselves to being shared and enjoyed in this manner. Social eating also means eliminating unhealthy distracters (such as having the television on and/or responding to calls and messages) so that you can engage your guests with stimulating conversation. Speaking of pleasant banter, this book provides the perfect mealtime topic—blending cooking, eating, and well-being!

Social eating means eliminating unhealthy distracters (such as having the television on and/or responding to calls and messages) so that you can engage your guests with stimulating conversation.

Shallot Frittatas

SERVES 6

These little baked omelets are a beautiful starter to an elegant meal or a lovely main course for a luncheon when paired with a green salad and some crusty bread. Easy enough to cook with kids or with people who have little or no cooking experience, frittatas can be a good confidence booster. You can also make a large one in a skillet to slice and share, but these individual sizes are lovely.

3 tablespoons unsalted butter
16 medium shallots, diced
Kosher salt, to taste
1 dozen large eggs, beaten

1 (8-ounce) package Boursin cheese, crumbled
¼ teaspoon freshly ground white pepper
Pinch ground nutmeg
2 tablespoons minced chives

Preheat the oven to 400°F. Grease 6 (½-cup) ramekins with nonstick spray and set them aside.

In a large nonstick skillet set over medium-high heat, melt the butter until the foaming subsides. Add the shallots, season with salt, and sauté until the shallots are tender and lightly golden brown. Transfer them to a large bowl to cool. Once the shallots have cooled, add the eggs, cheese, pepper, and nutmeg to the bowl, stirring gently until well combined. Divide the mixture evenly among the prepared ramekins, making sure that each has shallot and cheese in it.

Transfer the ramekins to a baking sheet and bake for 12 to 15 minutes, until the tops feel just firm.

Remove from the oven and let the frittatas rest for 5 minutes. Invert the ramekins onto plates, garnish with the chives, and serve.

Celery-Root Velouté with Crispy Sunchokes

SERVES 6

A velouté is a very smooth cream-based soup thickened slightly with flour, which can be a good technique to use for soups in general. Since this recipe involves both the soup part and the crispy garnish, it can be a great recipe to make with a partner. With everyone's busy schedules, it has become harder to focus on quality family time over the dinner table. Adding a starter like this soup can add a good 15 or 20 minutes to your meal, slowing you all down and giving you more time to be together.

6 small sunchokes, scrubbed and cut into ¼-inch slices

1 tablespoon extra virgin olive oil

Kosher salt and freshly ground black pepper, to taste

6 cups homemade or store-bought low-sodium chicken stock

4 tablespoons unsalted butter

4 shallots, minced

¼ cup all-purpose flour

3 pounds celery root (2–3 roots), peeled and roughly chopped

2 cups half and half

⅛ teaspoon ground nutmeg

Preheat the oven to 400°F. Grease a 10 × 14-inch baking sheet with nonstick spray and set it aside.

In a small bowl, toss together the sunchokes and oil until well coated. Arrange the sunchokes in a single layer on the prepared baking sheet. Season with salt and pepper. Roast for 15 to 20 minutes, until well browned and crispy. Set aside.

In a medium saucepan set over medium-high heat, bring the chicken stock to a simmer. In a heavy stockpot set over medium-low heat, melt the butter until it stops foaming. Add the shallots and sauté, stirring frequently, for 2 minutes, until they are translucent. Sprinkle the flour over the shallots and cook, stirring constantly, until everything melds together. Continue to cook for 2 minutes; this will remove the raw taste from the flour.

Remove the pot from the heat and whisk in 1 cup of the simmering stock, stirring very vigorously so that it smoothly combines with the shallot mixture and there are no lumps. When the mixture is smooth, stir in the rest of the stock.

Return the pot to the heat. Add the celery root, half and half, and nutmeg, stirring to combine. Increase the heat to medium-high and bring to a gentle boil. Reduce the heat to low and simmer, stirring occasionally, for 30 minutes, until the broth has thickened slightly and the celery root is very tender and can be mashed easily with the back of a spoon. Remove from the heat.

Using an immersion blender, purée the soup in the pot until it is extremely smooth and velvety. (Alternatively, purée the soup in batches in a regular blender.) Taste and add salt and pepper as needed.

Ladle into bowls, garnish with crispy sunchoke chips, and serve.

Celery, Green Apple, and Parmesan Salad

SERVES 8

The legendary writer and consummate hostess Nora Ephron said that the key to a great dinner party menu is to include at least one surprising element. It is a terrific conversation starter: whether it is a dish that you make because you ate it on a favorite vacation, or it was first cooked for you by a friend or family member, bringing a story to the dinner table can get the ball rolling. With that in mind, it is time to get out of your salad rut! This is a classic, but little-known, Italian salad—one of those dishes where simplicity belies a perfect flavor combination. Be sure to use the best quality Parmigiano-Reggiano here, as the cheese is not a garnish but a key ingredient in the salad.

2 heads celery
2 Granny Smith apples, cored, halved, and
    sliced thin
½ pound Parmigiano-Reggiano shavings,
    divided

Freshly squeezed juice of 1 lemon
¼–⅓ cup extra virgin olive oil
Kosher salt and freshly ground black pepper,
    to taste

Remove the bottom inch of the celery heads and separate the stalks. Rinse under cold water to remove any dirt and dry with paper towels. Trim off and discard the tops, and slice the stalks into ¼-inch-thick slices on a very strong diagonal to make them pretty. You want to slice across so that you slice through the strings, so that the celery is easier to eat.

In a large bowl, combine the celery, apple, and ⅓ pound of the cheese (two-thirds of the total quantity). Add the lemon juice and olive oil. Taste and add salt and pepper as needed. Garnish with the remaining ⅙ pound of cheese and serve.

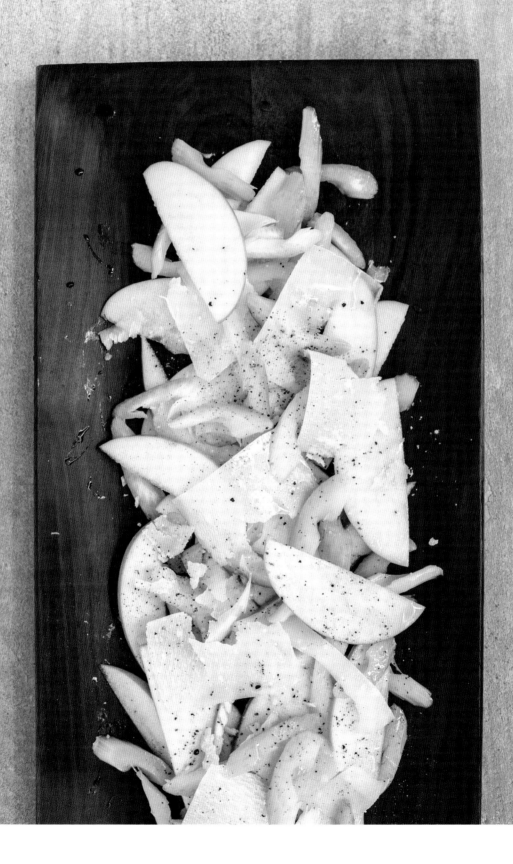

Sautéed Skate with Parsley Purée

SERVES 6

Very few of us eat enough fish in our diets. And when it comes to cooking for friends or loved ones, people can get into a fish rut, with the usual suspects of salmon, tuna, and halibut in heavy rotation. But if you have a good fishmonger, skate is a beautiful addition and will make your dining companions feel very spoiled. Since fish is very much a cook-at-the-last-minute dish, this is a great opportunity to cook with a partner, who can be focused on side dishes while you make the fish. This sort of teamwork can really be a good way to connect; the feeling of dividing and conquering for a larger good is bonding. It can also be a good way to make inroads with a teenager with whom you are having complicated communication issues. By assigning side-dish tasks and then allowing the teen to simply execute, you take the pressure off of the situation but still provide an opportunity for him or her to ask questions or solicit advice. If you cannot get skate, this recipe works well with sole or other flaky, mild fishes.

1 tablespoon kosher salt, plus more to taste
1 large bunch fresh flat-leaf parsley
1 teaspoon lemon zest, plus more for garnish
1 tablespoon freshly squeezed lemon juice
Pinch cayenne pepper (optional)

3 tablespoons extra virgin olive oil, plus more
   for garnish
Freshly ground black pepper, to taste
6 (8-ounce) skate fillets
2 tablespoons canola oil, divided
3 tablespoons minced chives, for garnish

Preheat the oven to 200°F.

In a medium bowl, make an ice bath with ice and cold water. Add the salt and stir until it dissolves. The water should taste salty like the sea. Set it aside.

Bring a small pot of salted water to a boil over medium-high heat. Using the stems of the parsley as a handle, swirl the leaves of the parsley in the water for 10 to 15 seconds, until the leaves are bright green. Plunge the parsley into the ice bath, swirling it until the parsley is no longer warm. Using a knife, remove and discard the stems. Transfer the leaves to a blender. Add ½ cup of the parsley cooking water, the lemon zest and juice, and the cayenne, if using. Pulse to combine. With the machine running on medium-high, drizzle in the olive oil until the mixture is smooth and creamy. Taste and add salt and pepper as needed. Set the parsley purée aside.

Season the fillets on both sides with salt and pepper. In a large nonstick skillet set over medium-high heat, heat 1 tablespoon of the canola oil until it shimmers. Slide 3 of the skate fillets into the pan and cook 3 to 4 minutes per side, until they are golden brown and cooked through. Transfer the skate to a shallow baking dish and keep them warm in the oven until ready to serve. Add the remaining tablespoon of canola oil to the skillet and repeat this process with the remaining pieces of skate.

Spread about 2 tablespoons of the parsley purée on each of 6 plates. Add a skate fillet on top, and garnish with olive oil, minced chives, and a light sprinkle of lemon zest. Serve hot.

Slow-Roasted Prime Rib

SERVES 6

Nothing is more special for an occasion than a standing rib roast. When you are connecting with a large group, a substantial roast is an easy way to impressively feed a big group of people. And since prime rib is something of a retro food, it can often spark some fun memories to share with the group, of parties or events from the past. But the last thing you want to do for your celebration is overcook a very expensive piece of beef! This recipe is pretty foolproof and very forgiving.

1 (4–5-pound) bone-in prime rib roast, room temperature (see Note)

Kosher salt and freshly ground black pepper, to taste

Preheat the oven to 200°F. Season the meat well on all sides with salt and pepper.

Place the roast on a rack in a roasting pan, transfer it to the oven, and cook for 2½ to 3 hours, until an instant-read thermometer inserted into the center of the roast registers 110°F.

Remove the roast from the oven and let rest for 30 minutes. Increase the oven temperature to 500°F. Transfer the roast back to the oven and continue cooking for 15 to 20 minutes, until an instant-read thermometer inserted into the center of the roast registers 130°F.

Remove the roast from the oven, transfer to a cutting board, tent with aluminum foil, and let it rest for 15 to 20 minutes before carving. To carve, remove the ribs in one piece, slice into 6 even slabs, and serve. Serve the ribs separately, or save for a cook's treat.

NOTE: Ask your butcher for a three-rib roast from the loin end.

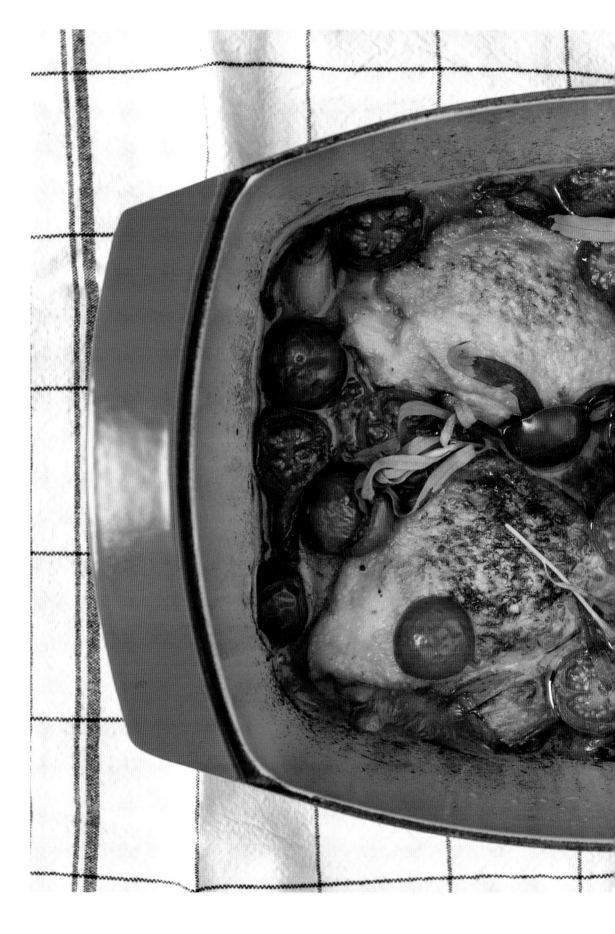

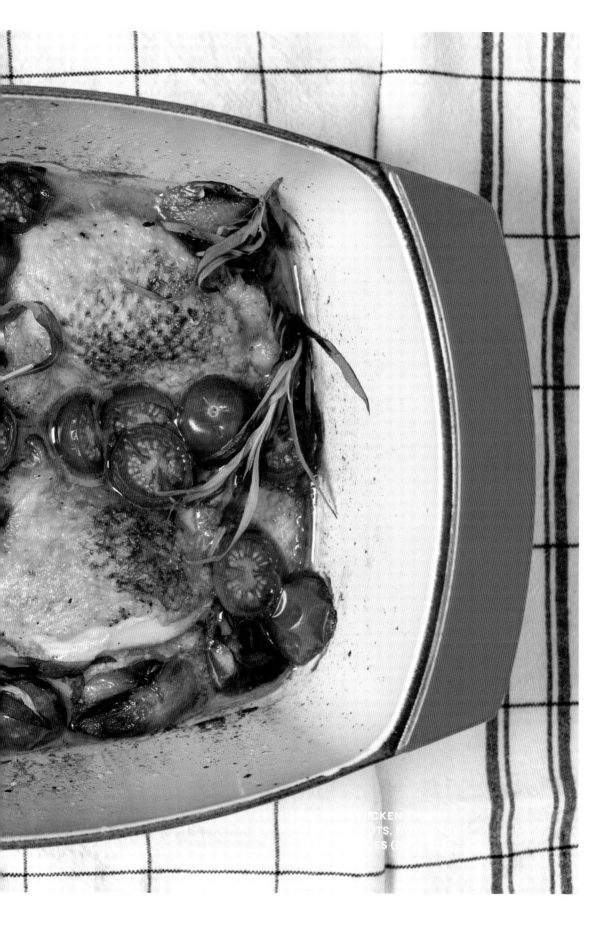

Braised Chicken Thighs with Shallots, Mushrooms, and Tomatoes

SERVES 4 TO 6

A few years ago, a braised chicken thigh recipe appeared in the *New York Times* by Andrew Zimmern. It contained an enormous amount of shallots and fresh tomatoes and a deeply flavored sauce. While the dish was quite wonderful just as it was, it required some last-minute work that was something of a hindrance for social cooking and entertaining. Since braised meat often tastes better the next day, this version of the dish can be almost completed the day before you want to serve it. Just reheat it gently in the oven. The addition of mushrooms makes it even more special, and the roasted tomatoes add even more punch than the fresh ones in the original recipe.

2 tablespoons all-purpose flour

1 tablespoon + 1 teaspoon kosher salt, divided, plus more to taste

½ tablespoon + ½ teaspoon freshly ground black pepper, divided, plus more to taste

8 bone-in, skin-on chicken thighs

1 tablespoon unsalted butter

2 teaspoons canola oil

12 medium shallots, halved

12 baby portobella or cremini mushrooms, cleaned and halved

2 cups white wine

2 tablespoons Dijon mustard

2 sprigs fresh tarragon

2 cups grape tomatoes, halved

2 tablespoons chopped fresh flat-leaf parsley, for garnish

1 tablespoon chopped fresh tarragon, for garnish

Preheat the oven to 300°F.

In a shallow baking dish, mix together the flour, 1 tablespoon of the salt, and ½ tablespoon of the pepper. Dredge each of the thighs in the flour mixture, pat to remove the excess flour, and set on a rack set over a baking sheet.

In a large Dutch oven set over medium-high heat, melt the butter until it stops foaming. Add the oil to increase the smoking point. Working in batches, add the thighs, skin-side down, and cook for 4 to 5 minutes per side, until the thighs are very golden brown. Transfer the thighs to a platter and set aside.

Add the shallots to the fat in the Dutch oven and toss to coat. Cook, flipping a couple of times, until the shallots are caramelized and softened, 10 to 12 minutes. If it seems that the shallots are in danger of burning, reduce the heat. Add the mushrooms and continue to cook for about 3 minutes, until they are a bit browned.

While the onions are browning, in a small bowl, combine the wine, the mustard, the remaining teaspoon of salt, and the remaining ½ teaspoon of pepper, stirring until the salt is dissolved. Pour the mixture into the Dutch oven. Add the thighs, nestling them among the shallots and mushrooms, so that the liquid in the pot comes about halfway up the sides of the chicken.

Tuck the tarragon sprigs in with the thighs and let the liquid come to a boil. Remove from the heat; cover the pot, transfer it to the oven, and cook for about 30 minutes. Remove the lid, remove and discard the tarragon sprigs, and scatter the tomatoes on top. Continue to cook, uncovered, for about 20 minutes.

Remove the pot from the oven and let the braised thighs cool for 1 hour. Cover the pot and store it in the fridge for up to 3 days.

The day you want to serve the thighs, remove the pot from the fridge and let it sit at room temperature for 1 hour. Preheat the oven to 350°F. In a small bowl, mix together the parsley and chopped tarragon.

Reheat the braised thighs in the oven, covered, for 30 minutes. Remove the lid and cook another 10 minutes, until the sauce has thickened and the tomatoes are well roasted.

Transfer the thighs to a serving platter. Taste the sauce and add salt and pepper as needed. If the sauce is not thick enough, put the pot over medium-high heat to reduce the sauce until it is the right consistency.

Pour the sauce, along with the shallots, mushrooms, and tomatoes, over the chicken. Garnish with the parsley and tarragon and serve.

Glazed Ham

Most people save ham for Thanksgiving, Christmas, or Easter, but it can be a festive choice all year round. One of the important things about cooking for larger social gatherings is to make sure you are cooking dishes that allow you to be a part of your party. A ham like this requires no last-minute fussing and no individual plating; it allows you to be a guest at your own gathering. The glaze takes it over the top!

Glaze
6 cloves garlic, minced
1 cup mango chutney
2 tablespoons ginger jam (see Note on
    page 197)
½ cup Dijon mustard
1 cup firmly packed light brown sugar

Zest of 1 orange
¼ cup freshly squeezed orange juice
1 tablespoon soy sauce

Ham
1 (10-pound) bone-in ham
1 cup water

To make the glaze, combine all of the ingredients in a small bowl and set aside.

To make the ham, trim off the skin, leaving ¼ to ½ inch of the fat. Score a diamond pattern into the first ¼ inch of flesh. (Your butcher can prep this for you if you are concerned, but it isn't difficult; just take your time.)

Preheat the oven to 350°F. Put the ham, fat-side up, in an 11 × 16-inch roasting dish. Add the water to the bottom. Cover the dish with aluminum foil.

Transfer to the oven and cook for 1 to 1½ hours, until an instant-read thermometer inserted into the thickest part of the meat registers 125°F to 130°F. Remove the foil and glaze the ham generously with the glaze. Return to the oven and cook, uncovered, for another 30 minutes.

Slice and serve hot or at room temperature.

Butterflied Leg of Lamb

While you can use this marinade on almost any meat, it is particularly wonderful with lamb. And lamb is a terrific dish for a small holiday celebration or dinner party.

Marinade
Juice and zest of 1 lemon
½ cup extra virgin olive oil
2 tablespoons Dijon mustard
1 tablespoon minced garlic
4 tablespoons fresh rosemary leaves
1 tablespoon soy sauce

1 tablespoon Worcestershire sauce
1 tablespoon red wine vinegar
1 teaspoon kosher salt
½ teaspoon freshly ground black pepper

Lamb
1 (3–4-pound) butterflied leg of lamb

To make the marinade, mix together all the marinade ingredients in a gallon-size zip-top bag.

To make the lamb, add it to the bag, press out as much air as possible, and smoosh the meat around to be sure that it is evenly coated with the marinade. Transfer the bag to the fridge and let the lamb marinate for at least 4 hours or as long as overnight.

Remove the bag from the fridge and set it aside for 40 minutes to bring the meat to room temperature. Meanwhile, preheat the oven to 400°F or prepare a grill.

Remove the lamb from the bag and discard the marinade; do not use it as a basting sauce.

If roasting, warm an ovenproof skillet over medium-high heat until a hand placed 2 inches over the surface can feel strong heat radiating from the pan. Place the lamb in the skillet and sear for 4 to 5 minutes per side, until the meat is well browned. Transfer the skillet to the oven and cook for 20 to 30 minutes, until an instant-read thermometer inserted into the thickest part of the lamb registers 135°F for medium rare.

If grilling, place the lamb over direct heat and grill for 10 to 12 minutes per side, until the meat is well seared. Reposition the lamb over indirect heat and cook for another 20 to 30 minutes, until an instant-read thermometer inserted into the thickest part of the lamb registers 135°F for medium rare.

Transfer the lamb to a carving board and let it rest for 15 minutes. Slice and serve hot.

Tomato Pudding

Potlucks are a wonderful way to bring people together. Sharing special dishes is what this whole chapter is about, so providing an opportunity for others to bring their own offerings not only takes the pressure off of the hosts but allows everyone to participate in bringing the group together. This savory take on a bread pudding is vegetarian friendly and a great side dish for almost any meat. It is usually a surprise for your guests, and a delicious one at that!

2 cups homemade or store-bought dried
   bread cubes
1 stick unsalted butter, melted
¾ cup firmly packed brown sugar
½ cup tomato paste
½ cup tomato purée

¼ cup freshly squeezed orange juice
Kosher salt and freshly ground black pepper,
   to taste
1 large beefsteak tomato or 3 Roma tomatoes,
   thinly sliced

Preheat the oven to 350°F.

In a medium (2-quart) casserole dish, toss the bread cubes and melted butter together to combine, then set aside.

In a medium saucepan set over medium-high heat, bring the brown sugar, tomato paste, tomato purée, and orange juice to a boil. Reduce the heat to medium-low and simmer for 5 minutes. Taste and add salt and pepper as needed.

Pour the hot mixture over the bread cubes. Arrange the tomato slices in a thin layer over the top. Sprinkle with salt.

Bake for 35 to 40 minutes, until the pudding is puffy and the corners of the bread cubes are browned. Cut the casserole into 6 squares and serve hot.

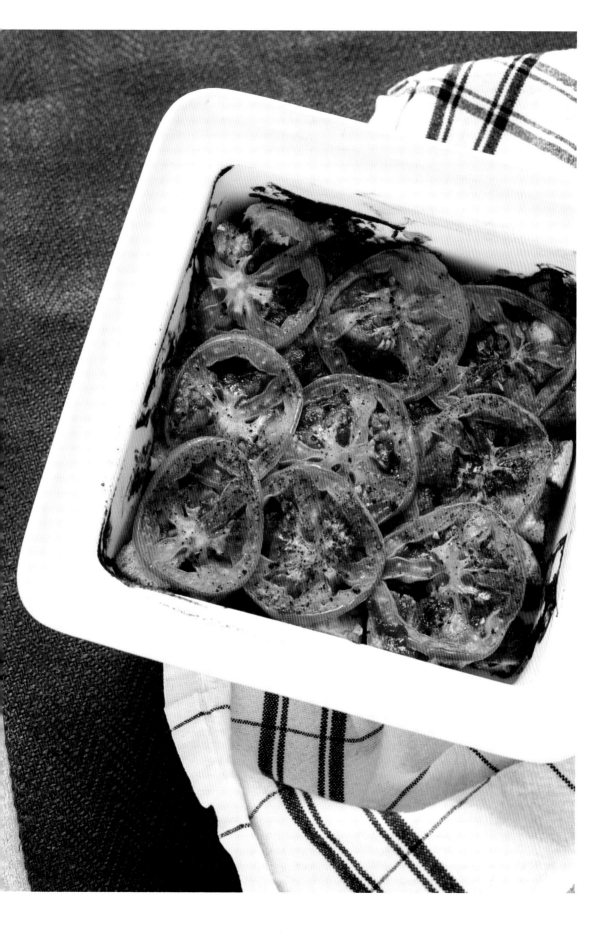

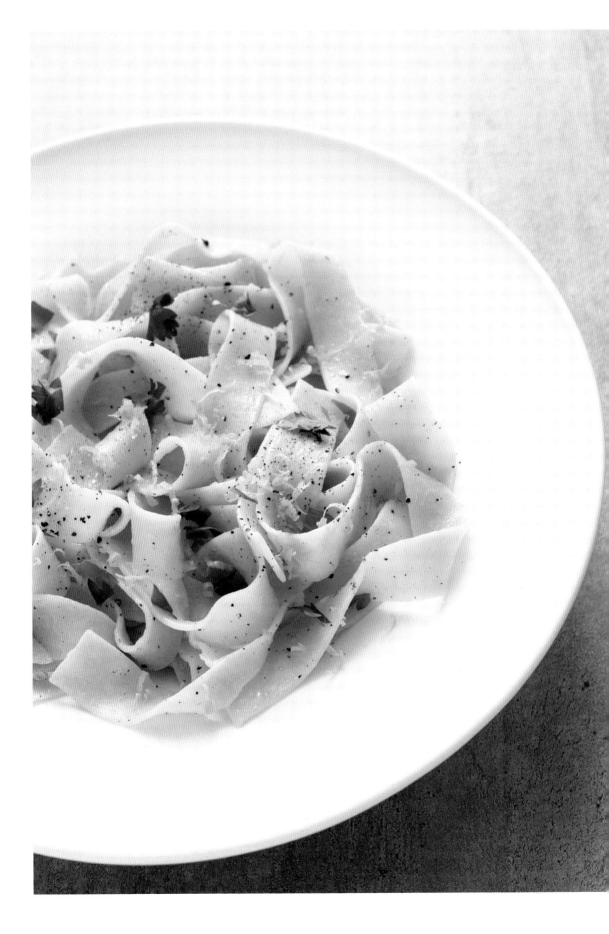

Truffled Pappardelle

This is one of those recipes you will turn to again and again. It comes together in a flash, so it is great for dinner parties when you want to spend time with your guests and not by yourself in the kitchen. It is terrific as a vegetarian entrée, too—just add a spoonful of softly scrambled eggs on top (I know, it sounds weird, but it tastes amazing!).

1 pound pappardelle or other wide, flat noodles
3½ ounces truffle butter, room temperature
3 tablespoons finely chopped chives or fresh
    flat-leaf parsley, divided

2 tablespoons lemon zest
Kosher salt and freshly ground black pepper,
    to taste

In a large pot of well-salted water, cook the pasta to al dente according to the package directions. Reserve ½ cup of the cooking water, drain the pasta, and return it to the pot, with the heat off. Stir in the truffle butter, 2½ tablespoons of the chives, and the lemon zest, mixing gently, so that everything is well incorporated but you don't break up the noodles.

Stir in the reserved cooking water, 1 tablespoon at a time, until the sauce is creamy and just coats the noodles without looking greasy. Taste and add salt and pepper as needed. The truffle butter and cooking liquid are salty, so you may not need extra salt.

Transfer the truffled pappardelle to a serving bowl, garnish with the remaining ½ tablespoon of chives, and serve.

Braised Broccolini

SERVES 4 TO 6 AS A SIDE

This is a great dish to make when you are entertaining, as you can arrange the ingredients in the pan up to 3 hours before you want to serve it. That way there is no fussing when your guests are there; you can stay present in the moment with them, and then just turn the stove on 15 to 20 minutes before you plan to serve dinner.

2 (8-ounce) packages broccolini, rinsed and drained (see Note)

1 cup homemade or store-bought low-sodium chicken stock

Kosher salt and freshly ground black pepper, to taste

2 tablespoons unsalted butter

In a medium sauté pan, arrange the broccolini in a single, even layer. Add the stock and season with salt and pepper. Put the butter in the center of the broccolini and cover the pan.

Turn the heat to high and cook, covered, for 15 minutes. You should see plenty of steam coming out of the sides of the lid. Lift the lid and check the liquid. Continue to cook, uncovered, until the liquid is almost completely gone and has become a light glaze.

Transfer to a platter and serve hot.

> **NOTE**: Broccolini, sometimes called broccolette or baby broccoli, is a cross between broccoli and Chinese broccoli. The stalks are skinny, the florets are looser than broccoli, and there is a better balance of sweet and bitter flavors—without the sulfurous smell or taste that can sometimes accompany broccoli.

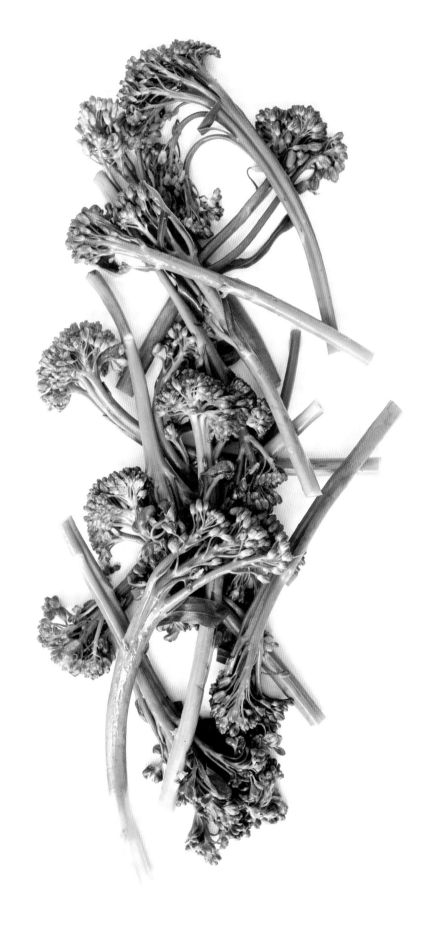

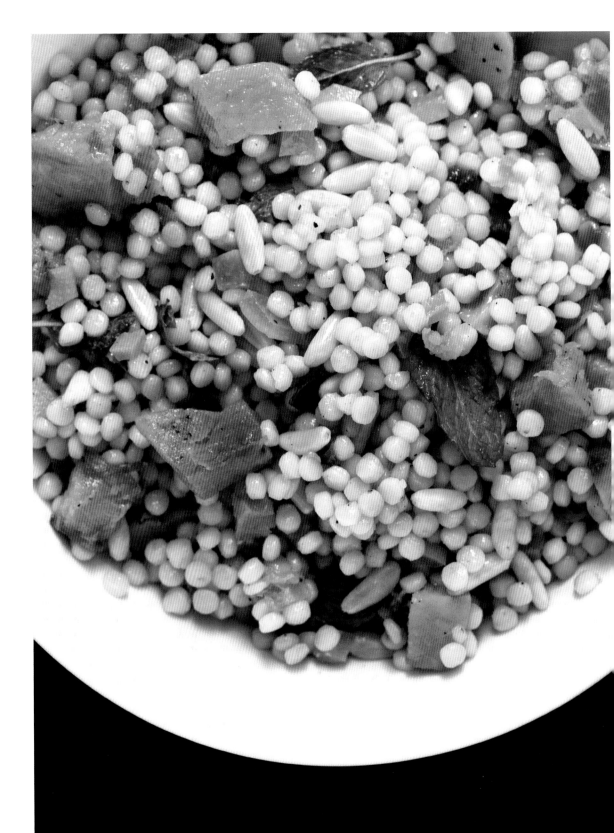

Israeli Couscous with Roasted Butternut Squash

SERVES 4 AS A SIDE

Israeli couscous is a small round pasta that makes a great basis for salads and side dishes. This recipe is terrific for vegetarians, beautiful to look at, and delicious when served both hot or cold. The original recipe from David Lebovitz called for preserved lemons, but those can be difficult to source, and besides, they added a bit of pickled, salted flavor that this bright and flavorful side dish doesn't need.

1 (1-pound) butternut squash, peeled and
    diced
2 tablespoons extra virgin olive oil, divided
1 teaspoon kosher salt, plus more to taste
1 large shallot, minced
Zest of 1 lemon
¼ cup golden raisins
¼ cup dried cherries, coarsely chopped
½ cup toasted pine nuts (see Note on page 159)

¼ teaspoon ground cinnamon
6 cups water
Pinch saffron threads
1 small stick cinnamon
1 cup Israeli couscous
Freshly ground black pepper, to taste
½ cup chopped fresh mint leaves, for garnish
    (small leaves can remain whole)

Preheat the oven to 400°F. Grease a baking sheet with nonstick spray and set aside.

In a medium bowl, toss together the squash and 1 tablespoon of the oil until well coated. Arrange the squash in a single, even layer on the prepared baking sheet and season with salt. Roast for about 20 minutes, until the squash is tender and browned. Remove from the oven, transfer to a large bowl, and set aside to cool.

In a large skillet set over medium-high heat, heat the remaining tablespoon of oil until it shimmers. Add the shallot and sauté until it is tender and lightly browned. Transfer the shallot to the bowl with the squash. Add the lemon zest, raisins, cherries, pine nuts, and ground cinnamon. Mix until fully combined, being gentle so that you don't mush up the squash.

In a large saucepan set over medium-high heat, combine the water, salt, saffron, and cinnamon stick and bring to a boil. Stir in the couscous and cook for 10 to 12 minutes, until it is al dente.

Drain the couscous well and discard the cinnamon stick. Transfer the couscous to the bowl with the rest of the ingredients; stir with a fork, as you would with rice, so that the couscous doesn't get gummy and clump together. Taste and add salt and pepper as needed.

Garnish with the mint and serve warm or at room temperature.

Chocolate–Hazelnut Cheesecake

SERVES 10 TO 12

Nothing says *party* like homemade cheesecake, and this version, which tastes like Nutella, takes it over the top. It is something of a mash-up of a crust I liked from an *Epicurious* cheesecake, paired with a simpler technique for filling that I preferred from a *Fine Cooking* cheesecake recipe, making for a new marriage that is simply delicious for any event. Plus, this is a great recipe to cook with a partner: one person can make the crust while the other works on the filling.

Crust

1 cup crushed Nabisco Famous Chocolate Wafers

1 ounce fine-quality bittersweet chocolate, grated

4 tablespoons unsalted butter, melted and cooled

Filling

3 (8-ounce) packages cream cheese, room temperature

1¼ cups granulated sugar

2 tablespoons all-purpose flour

1 teaspoon instant espresso powder

Pinch kosher salt

1 tablespoon pure vanilla extract

4 large eggs, room temperature

1½ cups Nutella, divided

⅓ cup chopped toasted hazelnuts, for garnish (see Note on page 159)

Preheat the oven to 300°F. Line a roasting pan with a folded cotton or linen towel and set aside. This will keep the cheesecake from sliding around in the pan.

To make the crust, in a small bowl, use a fork to mix together the crushed wafers, chocolate, and butter until combined. Transfer the mixture to a springform pan, pressing it into an even layer. Wrap the outside of the springform pan with a large piece of aluminum foil, place it in the prepared roasting pan, and set aside.

Put a kettle of water on to boil.

To make the filling, in a stand mixer fitted with the paddle attachment, beat the cream cheese on medium speed until fluffy and smooth. (Alternatively, you can use a large bowl and an electric handheld mixer.) In a small bowl, mix together the sugar, flour, espresso powder, and salt. Add the sugar mixture to the cream cheese and mix on medium speed until it is well blended and the sugar is no longer gritty. With the machine running, add the vanilla, and then 1 egg at a time, mixing each in completely before adding the next. Fold in ¾ cup of the Nutella until the filling is well mixed.

To assemble, pour the filling into the crust. Transfer the cheesecake, still on the roasting pan, to the middle rack of the oven. Pour the hot water from the kettle into the roasting pan so that the water dampens the towel and comes about halfway up the side of the springform pan. Bake for 55 to 65 minutes, until the center wobbles just slightly when you remove it from the oven.

Let the cheesecake cool in the pan, in the water, for 10 minutes, then transfer the springform pan carefully to a rack and let it cool completely before removing the springform side. Cover the cheesecake with plastic wrap and transfer it to the fridge. If the cake is not completely cooled when you do this, it will form condensation on the top underneath the plastic wrap.

Chill the cake for at least 3 hours or as long as overnight. Remove from the fridge and remove the plastic wrap. In a small microwave-safe bowl, warm the remaining ¾ cup of Nutella in the microwave for 30 seconds, or until it is just pourable. Spread the warm Nutella on the top of the chilled cheesecake and return it to the fridge for 1 hour.

Garnish with the hazelnuts. Slice and serve.

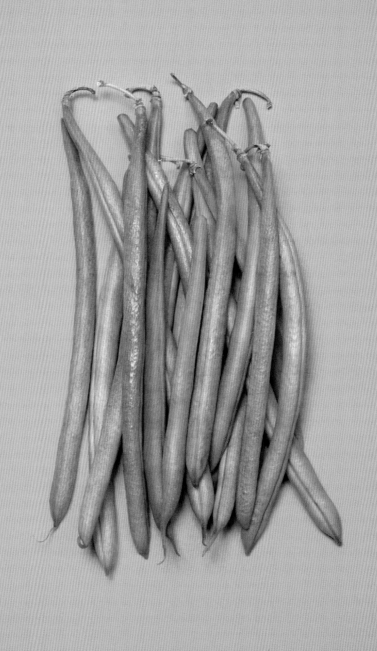

CHAPTER 9: Occupational Wellness

OCCUPATIONAL WELLNESS IS ABOUT **WORKING**. As is the case with many other wellness dimensions, this can be looked at as a continuum of sorts. Consider the following: unemployed, underemployed, unhappily employed, job, career, and vocation. Everyone falls somewhere on this spectrum, and your occupational well-being is as important as every other dimension. It begs an important question: Do you live to work or work to live? Regardless of your choice, cooking and eating can significantly support your work-related goals! Part of this involves eating at work. Many of us now eat both breakfast and lunch at work, not to mention eat at work-related social events. Interestingly enough, for many people, eating well seems to be easy at home, but then things go sideways at work. Some of this can be stress related, as food is a comfort when things get intense. Sometimes it's because the food we eat during our workdays is unsatisfying, sending us in search of quick fixes, often at a vending machine. Or, it can be difficult when colleagues seem to always be bringing in special treats and temptations. Being conscious of how your cooking and eating impact your occupational life can make a real differ-ence. What sort of fuel do you need to get through your day? Can shaking up your work dining options help you be more productive? Will having healthy, thoughtful snacks available to you at work help you avoid sugary, carb-laden, or processed-food temptations? And are there ways to participate in office pot-lucks and parties in a meaningful way, bringing in things that are delicious and homemade instead of just picking something up at the store?

COOKING for your occupational well-being is about efficiency and effectiveness. Preparing your foods well in advance of your workday—as much as a week ahead of time—will help reduce the morning scramble. Consider using the weekend to prepare your meals for the next three to five days. Some of the recipes in this chapter can be frozen and thawed later, while others have a longer shelf life. Pack lots of small portions of your favorites as snacks, instead of fewer large ones, so you can healthfully graze through-out the day. You can even pack a couple of extras—more than you might think you'll eat. Those who do are less likely to fall victim to the often-costly temptations found in vending machines or at local fast-food restaurants. Plus, you'll eat better, too!

EATING for your occupational well-being should be a priority. Think about how many hours you spend at work and how many food choices you have to make during those work hours. I've provided the perfect combination of easy recipes for you, and if you are so inclined, for your coworkers, too. Consuming smaller portions of your favorites in this chapter will help stabilize your blood sugar and consequently your energy levels. If you are one of the many people who experience that three o'clock slump, you might find that eating more protein at lunch and having energy-boosting snacks at your desk will help you more than a caffeinated beverage. When it comes to eating a primary meal—like lunch—step away from your desk! Though snacking while working is often acceptable, taking an eating break is the perfect way to nurture your overall wellness. If you are feeling like feeding your social well-being, too, then invite someone to share in your break with you. If you need quiet time, then make the great escape to a common area, to a park, or even to your car. We've also included recipes that could be shared with your coworkers in a meeting or perhaps left in a break room with a nice little note encouraging everyone to enjoy! We all know how much people appreciate the gift of food—and will appreciate you for your generosity. Eat smart, work smart, and live well.

When it comes to eating a primary meal—like lunch—step away from your desk!

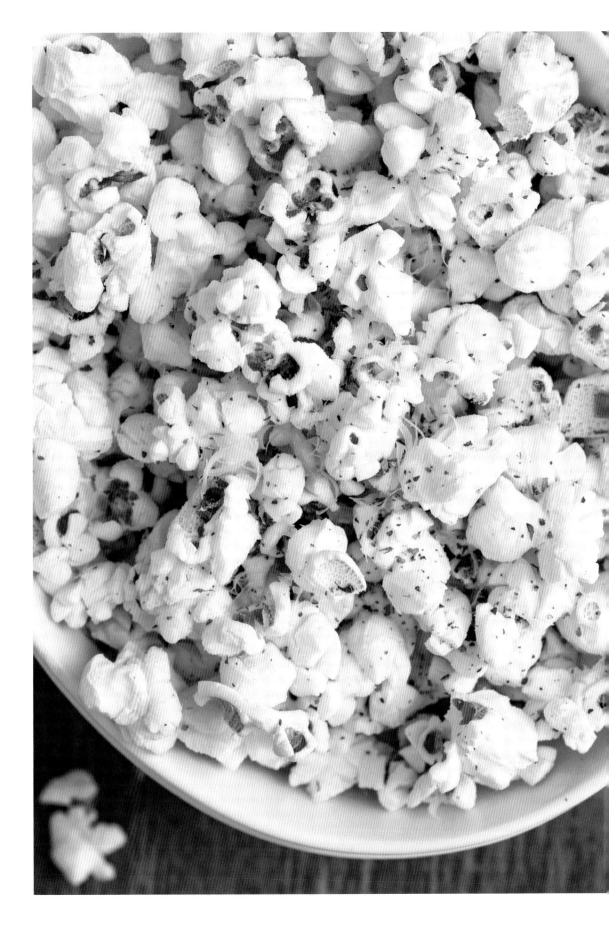

Homemade Microwave Seasoned Popcorn

SEASONING MIX SERVES ABOUT 18, POPCORN SERVES 2

When you need a snack at work, unhealthy options abound. Popcorn can seem like an easy choice, but the traditional store-bought packets are full of preservatives, salt, and fake fats. These homemade microwave popcorn packets can be made in an instant and taken to work, and the seasoning mix can live in your desk until you want to liven things up! This recipe serves two, so it is perfect for sharing.

Seasoning Mix
6 tablespoons nutritional yeast (see Note)
2 teaspoons ground mustard powder
1 tablespoon kosher salt, plus more to taste
2 teaspoons dried thyme leaves, herbes de Provence, or Italian herb mix

1 teaspoon garlic powder
½ teaspoon cayenne pepper (optional)

Popcorn Packet
½ cup popcorn kernels
1 tablespoon peanut oil
½ teaspoon kosher salt

To make the seasoning mix, in a small bowl combine all of the ingredients (add as much salt as desired). Transfer to an airtight container and store at room temperature until ready to use, up to 6 months.

To make the popcorn packet, in a small bowl combine the ingredients and mix well. Transfer to a plain brown-paper lunch bag. Fold the top of the bag over twice to make sure it is well sealed. The packet will last 24 hours at room temperature or up to a week in the fridge.

Microwave the popcorn on high for 3 minutes, or until the popping slows to 1 or 2 seconds between pops. Be careful when opening the bag, as the escaping steam will be hot.

Sprinkle about 1 tablespoon of the seasoning mix into the bag and shake around. Pour into a bowl and serve.

> **NOTE**: You can find nutritional yeast with the dietary supplements or bulk foods at Whole Foods or any health-food store. While it sounds like a strange addition, it has a nutty flavor that is reminiscent of Parmesan and pairs great with popcorn. If you can't find it, you can substitute grated Parmesan, but this will mean you will have to store the mix in the fridge for no longer than 3 days.

Spiced Almonds

SERVES 8

Almonds, high in protein, are a terrific source of quick energy when you are deskbound. This spicy version is easy to make and less boring than just plain nuts. You can keep a jar of them in your desk for when your energy starts to flag.

2 teaspoons extra virgin olive oil
1 teaspoon ground cumin
¼ teaspoon garlic powder
¼ teaspoon cayenne pepper

½ teaspoon kosher salt
¼ teaspoon ground mustard powder
¼ teaspoon fish sauce
2 cups whole raw almonds

In a nonstick skillet set over medium-low heat, heat the oil until it shimmers. Add the cumin, garlic powder, cayenne, salt, and mustard powder and stir for about 30 seconds. Add the fish sauce and stir to combine. Add the almonds and cook, stirring, until they are well coated.

Remove from the heat, transfer to a baking sheet in one layer, and let cool. Transfer the almonds to an airtight container and store at room temperature for up to 1 week.

Gazpacho

I think of this summery soup as a savory smoothie and was excited to find a version of this recipe from NPR. You can drink it right out of a thermos if you are in a rush, or pour it into a bowl and garnish it with croutons and crumbled goat cheese or feta if you have more time. It is low calorie, so you can add a sandwich on the side if you are so inclined. I choose not to strain this version, so you get all the benefits of the vegetables' fiber to help fill you up. This is also a great reminder about being adaptable: if you like the flavor of the soup but don't like the texture this way, you can strain it. Make it over the weekend and portion it out throughout the workweek.

12 ripe plum tomatoes, diced
2 medium seedless cucumbers, peeled and cut
   into chunks
1 large red bell pepper, seeded and cut into
   chunks
2 small shallots, minced
1 clove garlic

1½ tablespoons sherry vinegar, plus more to
   taste
2 tablespoons homemade or store-bought low-
   sodium vegetable stock
1 cup extra virgin olive oil
Kosher salt and freshly ground black pepper,
   to taste

Put the tomatoes, cucumbers, bell pepper, shallots, garlic, vinegar, and stock in a blender. Pulse several times until the mixture becomes a chunky paste. Turn the blender to medium-high speed and slowly drizzle in the olive oil until the mixture is smooth. Taste and add salt, pepper, and vinegar as needed.

Serve at room temperature or slightly chilled.

> **NOTE:** If you make this soup ahead of time, be sure to leave it out at room temperature for at least one hour before serving, as the olive oil will solidify in the fridge and create little pockets of oil that aren't very tasty. Just give it a good shake or another whiz in the blender before serving.

Mason Jar Salad

The difference between my mason jar salad and most others is that I eschew lettuce. A salad for lunch doesn't satisfy for very long if it is mostly lettuce. If you love lettuce, I recommend storing it separate from the salad. Before eating, shake up the mason jar salad and then serve it on a bed of the lettuce. I encourage you to try it without lettuce, though, as it is much more satisfying. You can make a week's worth of jars at once, which makes planning lunches for work a snap. Once you learn the method, you can make endless variations, which means you'll never get into a lunch rut.

¼ cup salad dressing of your choice
⅓ cup canned chickpeas, rinsed, drained, and dried
⅓ cup halved grape tomatoes
⅓ cup chopped cucumbers
⅓ cup diced zucchini or yellow squash
⅓ cup grated carrots

⅓ cup cooked quinoa, wheat berries, or brown rice
1 tablespoon chopped fresh herbs, such as parsley, chives, dill, or basil
2 tablespoons sunflower seeds or sliced almonds

Put the dressing in a 1-quart mason jar. Add the chickpeas, tomatoes, cucumbers, zucchini, carrots, and quinoa, in that order. Top the salad with the fresh herbs and sunflower seeds.

Seal the jar and store it in the fridge until ready to use, up to 5 days. To serve, shake the jar until all the ingredients are well combined.

NOTE: For more protein, add some diced chicken or a can of dried tuna flakes before you shake. You can also pack garnishes—like olives, crumbled or shredded cheeses, or croutons—separately.

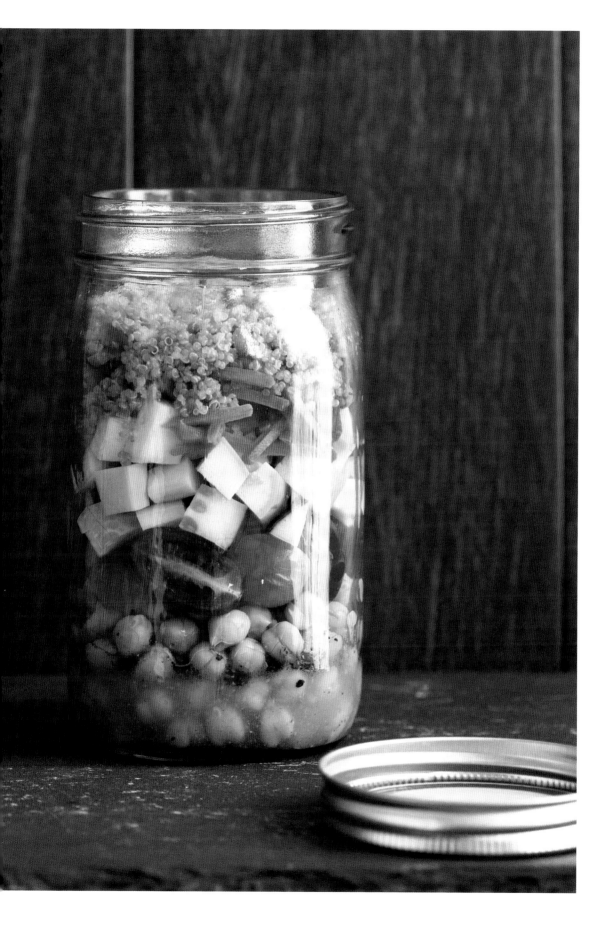

Desktop Niçoise with Anchovy Vinaigrette

SERVES 4

Classic niçoise salad is usually presented on a large platter, which makes it a beautiful luncheon dish but not so convenient for a workplace lunch. I've turned it into a chopped salad—easy to eat and no less delicious. I prefer a more rustic vinaigrette for this salad. If you want a smoother texture, make the vinaigrette in a blender or food processor. This dressing announces its presence in a wonderful way. It is so delicious that this recipe makes much more than you need, so that you can find other uses for it! It is great on any type of salad but also terrific as a dip for crudités, a sauce for fish, or a marinade for chicken or lamb. It will keep for a week in the fridge.

1 pound baby red or yellow potatoes, halved
1 pound green beans, trimmed and cut into
    1-inch pieces
4 (5-ounce) cans tuna packed in olive oil
2 tomatoes, chopped into 1-inch chunks
1 cucumber, peeled, seeded, and chopped into
    1-inch chunks

½ cup pitted and halved niçoise or Kalamata
    olives
⅓ cup Anchovy Vinaigrette (recipe follows),
    plus more as needed
Kosher salt and freshly ground black pepper,
    to taste
4 hard-boiled eggs, quartered, for garnish
8 anchovy fillets (optional), for garnish

In a medium pot place the potatoes and add cold water until the potatoes are covered by 1 inch. Salt the water well and bring to a boil over medium-high heat, then cook for 16 to 20 minutes, until the potatoes are fork tender. Add the green beans to the pot for just the last minute of cooking, then drain the potatoes and beans together and let rest in the strainer to dry completely.

Drain the tuna and flake it into a large bowl. Add the green beans, potatoes, tomatoes, cucumbers, and olives, tossing to mix. Add the vinaigrette. Taste and add salt, pepper, and more vinaigrette as needed.

Divide the salad between 4 airtight containers. Garnish each with 4 quarters of hard-boiled egg and 2 anchovy fillets, if using. Transfer the portions to the fridge and store until needed, up to 3 days.

Anchovy Vinaigrette

½ cup freshly squeezed lemon juice
4 large shallots, finely minced
½ teaspoon kosher salt
½ teaspoon freshly ground black pepper
6 tablespoons Dijon mustard
3 tablespoons anchovy paste
3 tablespoons capers, chopped
1½ cups extra virgin olive oil

In a small bowl, mix together the lemon juice and shallots. Let sit for 10 minutes to take the harsh bite out of the shallots. Add the salt and pepper, stirring until the salt is dissolved. Add the mustard, anchovy paste, and capers and stir until well blended. While stirring the mixture with a spatula or fork, slowly add the oil. With this amount of mustard, the dressing will practically emulsify itself; you don't need to whisk it. If the dressing isn't fully combined, pour it into a large jar or container with a lid that seals well and give it a good shake.

Store in the fridge until ready to use, up to 1 week. Let it come to room temperature and shake it again before using.

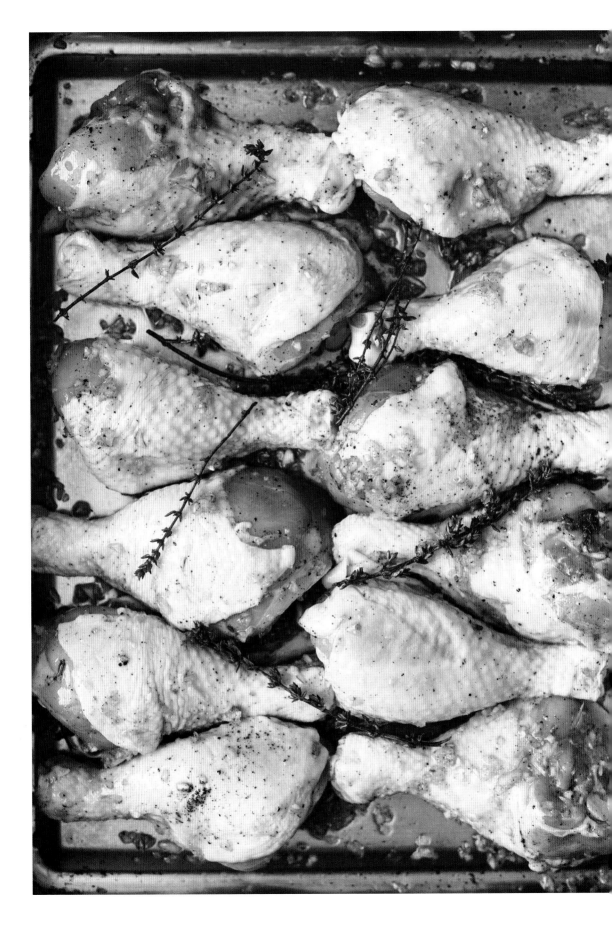

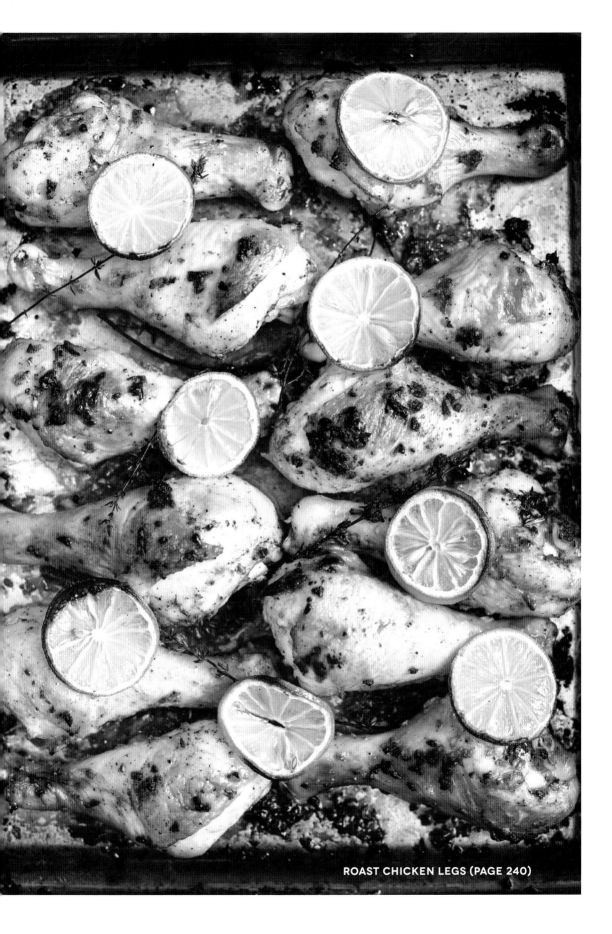

ROAST CHICKEN LEGS (PAGE 240)

Roast Chicken Legs

SERVES 8 AS AN ENTRÉE OR 16 AS A PART OF A BUFFET

Chicken legs are great for work or school lunches because they are a classic one-handed food. But it never occurred to me to just make the legs by themselves until I saw a version of this recipe in an old issue of *Gourmet Magazine*. And if you are having a work event, they are an inexpensive and easy way to feed a crowd. This recipe will take care of everyone in your family for a couple of lunches, or it will be a great addition to a workplace potluck.

4 tablespoons canola oil
4 tablespoons chopped shallot
1½ tablespoons pure maple syrup
2 teaspoons soy sauce
1 teaspoon kosher salt
½ teaspoon freshly ground black pepper

½ teaspoon red pepper flakes
2 tablespoons fresh thyme leaves
1 teaspoon smoked paprika
2 lemons, sliced thinly
16 chicken drumsticks

Preheat the oven to 450°F. Line a 10 × 14-inch baking sheet with aluminum foil and grease with nonstick spray.

In a large bowl, mix together the oil, shallot, maple syrup, soy sauce, salt, black pepper, red pepper flakes, thyme, paprika, and lemon slices. Add the chicken legs and toss to coat well. Divide the chicken legs and lemon slices between 2 gallon-size zip-top bags. Add any leftover sauce evenly between the bags. Press out as much air as possible, seal the bags, and let them sit at room temperature for 30 minutes to 1 hour. Arrange the marinated legs on the prepared baking sheet so that they are alternating head to toe and touching as little as possible. Scatter the lemon slices on top of the legs.

Bake for 25 to 35 minutes, until the skin is crispy and browned and an instant-read thermometer inserted into the thickest part of the meat (but not touching the bone) registers 165°F.

Remove the chicken legs from the oven and let them rest for 10 to 15 minutes. Serve warm or at room temperature.

> **NOTE:** If you are taking these to a work function and want to serve them warm, reheat them in a 350°F oven for 18 to 20 minutes. If your work does not have a large enough fridge, you can freeze the legs the night before and take them out in the morning; they will be thawed at room temperature by the time lunch rolls around.

Satay Root Vegetables

Vegetarians can have a tough time of it in the workplace, with lunch options often consisting of an endless series of bland salads. This Thai-inspired dish is easy to pull together, delicious hot or cold, and, when served over basmati rice, a filling and healthy meatless lunch. The peanut sauce is also great with grilled tofu.

1 large sweet potato, peeled and cut into 8 wedges
2–3 large carrots, peeled and cut into 2-inch chunks
2–3 large parsnips, peeled and cut into 2-inch chunks

2 tablespoons canola oil
Kosher salt and freshly ground black pepper, to taste
Peanut Sauce, for serving (recipe follows)

Preheat the oven to 400°F.

In a large bowl, toss together the sweet potato, carrots, parsnips, and oil. Season well with salt and pepper. Arrange on a rimmed baking sheet in a single layer and roast, flipping once, for 35 to 40 minutes, until the veggies are tender in the middle and crispy and browned outside.

Serve hot with the peanut sauce.

Peanut Sauce

1 teaspoon grated fresh ginger
1 teaspoon dark agave syrup
1 teaspoon ground cumin
1 tablespoon soy sauce
1 tablespoon dark sesame oil
2 tablespoons canola oil

2 tablespoons rice vinegar
Pinch red pepper flakes
½ cup natural no-stir creamy peanut butter
Kosher salt and freshly ground black pepper, to taste

In a medium bowl, mix together the ginger, agave syrup, cumin, soy sauce, sesame oil, canola oil, vinegar, and red pepper flakes until combined. Slowly fold in the peanut butter. (The peanut butter should incorporate smoothly.) If the sauce is too stiff, add hot tap water, 1 tablespoon at a time, until you get the right consistency. Taste and add salt and pepper as needed.

Transfer to an airtight container and store in the fridge until ready to use, up to 5 days. Bring to room temperature and stir well before using.

Roast-Beef Sandwich with Horseradish Cream and Pickled Onions

SERVES 1

I wanted to give you this recipe to use with either deli roast beef or leftover roast beef or sliced steak—something with a little more oomph than your usual sandwich. This protein-packed sandwich will fill you up at lunch and keep your energy up, and it is perfect for those days when you know you won't be able to leave your desk. Just because you are busy and don't have time to focus on a knife-and-fork lunch doesn't mean you don't deserve something special. If you are making lunches for the whole family, the pickled onion and horseradish cream recipes make plenty for a crowd; all you need is more bread and meat!

Horseradish Cream
½ **cup heavy cream**
1 **cup sour cream**
1 **tablespoon freshly grated horseradish**
Zest of 1 lemon
1 **teaspoon freshly squeezed lemon juice**
2 **tablespoons minced chives**

Kosher salt and freshly ground black pepper, to taste

Assembly
1 **soft bun or 2 slices sourdough bread**
Pickled Onions (recipe follows), to taste
4 **ounces thinly sliced roast beef**
1 **generous handful arugula**

To make the horseradish cream, in a chilled bowl whip the cream into soft peaks with an electric handheld mixer. Fold in the sour cream. Add the horseradish, lemon zest and juice, and chives, mixing to combine. Taste and add salt and pepper as needed. Transfer to an airtight container and store in the fridge until ready to use, up to 5 days. This sauce is delicious on all sorts of meats and fish, and even vegetables!

To assemble the sandwich, spread a generous amount of the horseradish cream on both sides of the bun or on the slices of bread. Add as many Pickled Onions as needed to the bottom slice. Add the roast beef on top and then the arugula. Finish with the top bread slice and wrap in aluminum foil or place in a zip-top bag, and store in the fridge until about 30 minutes before you want to eat. Letting the sandwich warm a bit at room temperature will bring out the flavors.

Pickled Onions

1½ cups white vinegar
6 tablespoons granulated sugar
½ teaspoon kosher salt
2 dried bay leaves
10 allspice berries
10 whole cloves
½ teaspoon red pepper flakes
2 large red onions, thinly sliced into rings

In a small saucepan set over medium heat, bring the vinegar, sugar, salt, bay leaves, allspice, cloves, and red pepper flakes to a boil. Add the onions and stir well to submerge the slices in the liquid. Remove the pan from the heat and let sit until the mixture has completely cooled. Transfer the onions, in their brine, to an airtight container and store in the fridge until ready to use, up to 2 weeks. Use in all sorts of sandwiches and salads.

> **NOTE:** While the onions will keep for several months in the fridge, they're best in the first week, when they are still nice and crisp. The longer they sit, the soggier they'll get.

BLT Baguette

If you are going to the trouble to make bacon over the weekend, it is always a good idea to make some extra to have on hand for this sandwich during the week!

1 tablespoon mayonnaise, plus more to taste
1 (6-inch) piece French baguette, halved
   lengthwise

4 slices ripe red and yellow tomato
4 slices thick-cut bacon, cooked until crisp
2 leaves Bibb lettuce

Spread the mayonnaise on both baguette halves. Shingle the tomatoes on the bottom slice and top with the bacon. Add the lettuce and close the sandwich. Wrap it tightly in plastic wrap to keep it compressed, and store in the fridge until ready to eat.

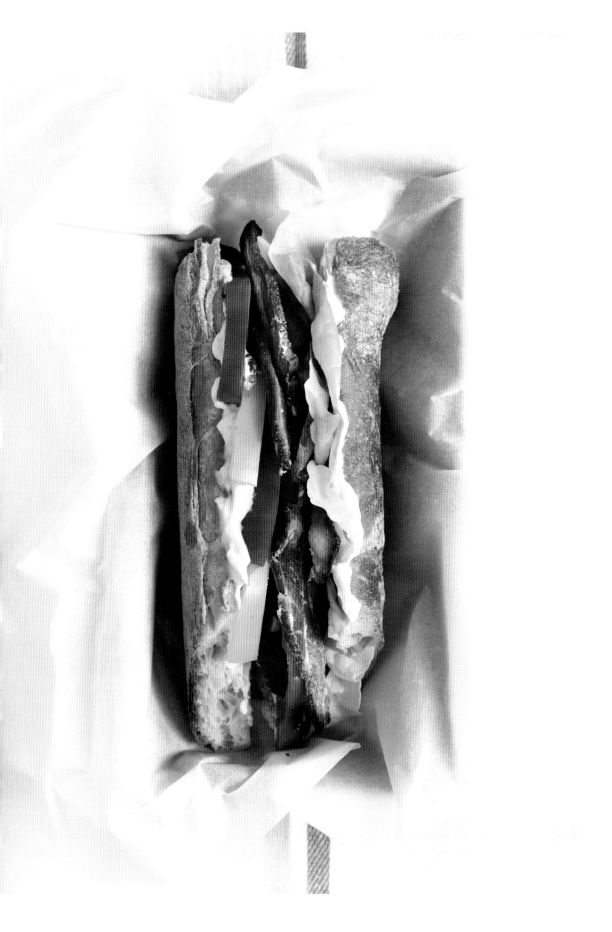

Spinach Pasta Salad

I never much liked pasta salads, finding them either swimming greasily in bottled Italian dressing or clumped with mayo. But, I saw a version of this recipe on *Serious Eats*, and when I gave it a try it flipped the script on pasta salad for me. This vibrant, green pasta salad replaces the usual mayonnaise-based dressing or vinaigrette with an olive tapenade. While you can make tapenade yourself, these days it is easy to find high-quality ones in the store, which makes this recipe even easier. If you want the challenge, find a great tapenade recipe and use ¾ cup of it for this recipe. This salad is easy to punch up with leftover chicken or turkey, a can of tuna, or any other leftover proteins you have lying around. But, because it has no meat, soft cheese, or mayo in it, this salad will keep in your fridge for up to five days, so you will get plenty of lunches out of it.

1 (6.5-ounce) jar green or black olive tapenade, such as Meditalia

½ cup chopped pitted mild green olives, like Cerignola

Zest of 1 lemon

3 quarts water

½ tablespoon kosher salt, plus more to taste

1 pound penne or other small pasta

¼ cup extra virgin olive oil

1 pound baby spinach leaves, washed and dried

½ cup grated Parmesan

Freshly ground black pepper, to taste

In a small bowl, mix together the tapenade, olives, and lemon zest and set aside.

In a large pot set over high heat, bring the water and salt to a boil. Stir in the penne and cook for 8 to 12 minutes, until al dente. Reserve ½ cup of the pasta water and drain the pasta.

Transfer the pasta to a large bowl. Stir in the olive oil and toss to coat. Add the tapenade mixture and stir until the pasta is well coated. Add the pasta water, 1 to 2 tablespoons at a time as needed to thicken; the dressing should just coat the pasta but not be soupy. Add the spinach, a couple of handfuls at a time, and let the still-warm pasta wilt the spinach slightly as you combine them. Add the Parmesan. Taste and add salt and pepper as needed.

Serve chilled or at room temperature.

Crudités with Buttermilk Dressing

This is a great snack that's easy to pack. Here I provide my favorite vegetable combination, a blend of crunchy veggies that are savory and a little sweet, but use whatever you love.

¼ cup Buttermilk Dressing (recipe follows)
1 cup 3-inch celery sticks
1 cup baby carrots

1 cup cauliflower florets
1 cup red bell pepper sticks

Pour 1 tablespoon of the dressing into each of 4 (½-pint) mason jars. Evenly divide the crudités into 4 portions, then stand them up in the dressing. Seal the jars and store them in the fridge until ready to eat. If you don't have mason jars for this, you can pack the crudités in zip-top sandwich bags and the dip in small airtight containers.

Buttermilk Dressing

MAKES ABOUT 1 CUP

¼ cup buttermilk
¼ cup mayonnaise
¼ cup sour cream
1 tablespoon water
1 tablespoon minced shallot
1 tablespoon minced fresh flat-leaf parsley

1 teaspoon minced chives
1 tablespoon freshly squeezed lemon juice
2 teaspoons minced fresh dill
½ teaspoon garlic powder
¼ teaspoon kosher salt
¼ teaspoon freshly ground black pepper

In a large bowl, mix together all of the ingredients until well combined. Transfer to an airtight container and store in the fridge until ready to use, up to 1 week. Serve cold.

Pizza Strudel

Offices can be tough places to have parties or events, especially if the kitchen isn't particularly well equipped. While this strudel is delicious hot, it is also perfectly great at room temperature, not to mention easy to make for a crowd. This strudel is great when served with your favorite marinara sauce.

1 pound sweet Italian sausage, removed from the casings

½ pound grated mozzarella

½ pound grated fontina or provolone

1 pound pizza dough (see Note)

½ pound pepperoni slices

2 tablespoons extra virgin olive oil

2 tablespoons grated Parmesan

Preheat the oven to 350°F. Grease a baking sheet and set aside.

In a medium nonstick skillet set over medium-high heat, cook the sausage for about 8 minutes, or until lightly browned, fully cooked with no pinkness, and well crumbled. Transfer the sausage to a plate lined with paper towels to drain. In a small bowl, mix the mozzarella and fontina and set aside.

Lightly flour a clean work surface and roll out the dough to an 11 × 14-inch rectangle. Cover the dough with the cheese, leaving 1 inch of dough around the edges. Sprinkle the crumbled sausage evenly over the cheese, and then do the same with the pepperoni. Starting on the long edge, roll the dough tightly around the filling to form a log, pinching the edges closed.

Transfer the roll, seam-side down, to the prepared baking sheet. Brush the outside of the roll with the olive oil and sprinkle evenly with the Parmesan.

Bake for 20 to 30 minutes, until the outside is golden brown and crisp and the inside is fully cooked. Transfer the strudel to a wire rack and let it cool for 10 minutes. Cut the strudel into 1-inch slices. Serve hot or at room temperature.

> **NOTE**: I recommend either buying premade dough, if your grocer carries it, or stopping into your favorite pizza place and asking to buy some from them. If you prefer to make homemade dough, use your favorite recipe.

Apple Cake with Chocolate Chips

SERVES 12

This easy cake is the perfect thing to bring to the office as a treat for your colleagues or as your contribution to the holiday buffet. It is dead easy, and while the combination of apples and chocolate might seem incongruous, it is absolutely delicious! Stacey's godmother shared the recipe, and it is one of my favorites.

2 cups all-purpose flour
2 cups granulated sugar
4 large eggs
1 cup vegetable oil
2 teaspoons ground cinnamon
1 teaspoon baking soda

1 tablespoon pure vanilla extract
Pinch kosher salt
3 large or 4 medium sweet and crisp apples, such as Fuji or Honeycrisp, cubed (about 4 cups)
1 cup semisweet chocolate chips

Preheat the oven to 325°F. Grease a 9 × 13-inch baking dish and set aside.

In a large bowl, combine the flour, sugar, eggs, oil, cinnamon, baking soda, vanilla, and salt. Add the apples and chocolate chips and stir well. Spread into the prepared pan. It will look like there is barely enough batter to coat the apple chunks and chocolate chips, but do not worry; it expands.

Bake for 40 to 45 minutes, until a skewer inserted into the middle of the cake comes out clean. Remove the cake from the oven and let it cool completely in the pan. Slice and serve.

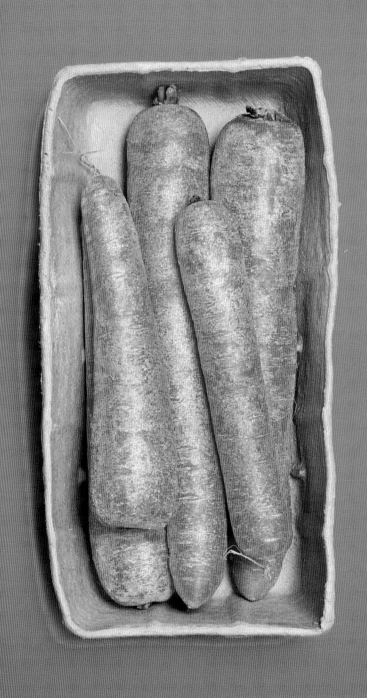

CHAPTER 10: Financial Wellness

FINANCIAL WELLNESS IS ABOUT **SPENDING**. We all have little control over the simple fact that we must spend in order to survive. However, we do have some level of control over how much we choose to spend and on what. And while some subscribe to the notion that when it comes to money, more is better, I'd suggest that it is not about how much you have, but how well you balance what you have. Research clearly shows that effective money management, rather than how much you earn, leads to happiness. From this perspective, those who choose to live within their means are the ones financially well-off. Wellness is about making those life choices that support our goals, and financial well-being is no exception!

COOKING for your financial well-being means purchasing ingredients that fit your food budget and that are a good quality for the price. It also means seeking out sales or buying ingredients in bulk when you are stocking up on things you use most. It means being mindful of buying the correct amount of perishable ingredients, so that you can use them up before they expire or go bad, and it means making thoughtful choices about managing leftovers. One way to do this is to connect with other like-minded cooks through social media to find the lowest-cost, highest-quality ingredients, which might mean exploring a CSA box from a local farmer or even going in with friends or family on buying a half of a cow or pig and dividing up the cuts between your freezers—a very cost-effective way of having access to meats, which are usually the most expensive component in a dish. But cooking for financial wellness can also mean exploring cuts of meats that are less expensive but no less delicious and satisfying when prepared well. It means growing your own produce if you are able and inclined. It means being thrifty in the kitchen and using up what is already in your pantry—things that might be an afterthought. The recipes that follow make delicious low-cost meals *and* take advantage of ingredients that you've probably got on hand but haven't used in a while.

EATING for your financial well-being means doing so in a manner that supports your financial goals. For example, if you aspire to save money like many of us, then consider eating less. This has positive implications for other wellness dimensions, too. By eating less, you not only save money but also reduce your caloric intake, which may support your weight-management goals and enhance your physical wellness. Many of these recipes will have slightly smaller portions. Eating less also means stabilizing your blood sugar and keeping your energy levels at their peak, which is great for intellectual wellness. However, if you are eating for pure indulgence, and your financial portfolio allows, then purchase and enjoy the highest-quality ingredients. And while many people routinely hire a personal trainer, consider hiring a personal chef, which surprisingly can cost about the same amount. Doing so may leave you with more time to focus on other areas of your well-being, which may prove a worthwhile investment.

When it comes to money, I'd suggest that it is not about how much you have, but how well you balance what you have.

Fromage Fort

Cheese is one of those things that I always seem to have too much of lying around. And when you get down to the little nubbins, it can be sad—not enough of a piece to serve, but too yummy to discard. The French, being both thrifty and devoted cheese lovers, have figured out a way to use up not only leftover bits of cheese but leftover wine as well! It looks prettier with white wine but tastes just as good if you use red. This dip is a delicious spread on slices of baguette, but it also makes for wonderful grown-up grilled cheese sandwiches.

½–¾ pound leftover cheese chunks (whatever you have lying around)
1 clove garlic

¼ cup leftover red or white wine
Kosher salt and freshly ground black pepper, to taste

Place the cheese, garlic, and wine in the bowl of a food processor and pulse until a smooth paste forms. Taste and add salt and pepper as needed. Transfer to an airtight container and store in the fridge until ready to use, up to 1 week.

Bottom-of-the-Jar Vinaigrettes

MAKES ABOUT ½ CUP

These salad dressings are a godsend. And while the results are always very different, the recipe is the same.

1 leftover jar mustard, jam, or honey
   (1–2 teaspoons, depending on the jar)
2 tablespoons vinegar of choice
6 tablespoons oil of choice

Generous pinch kosher salt, plus more as
   needed
Pinch freshly ground black pepper, plus more
   as needed

To the mustard jar, add the vinegar, oil, salt, and pepper. Shake the dickens out of it. Taste and add salt and pepper as needed. Seal the jar and store in the fridge until ready to use, up to 1 week. Bring back to room temperature and shake well before using.

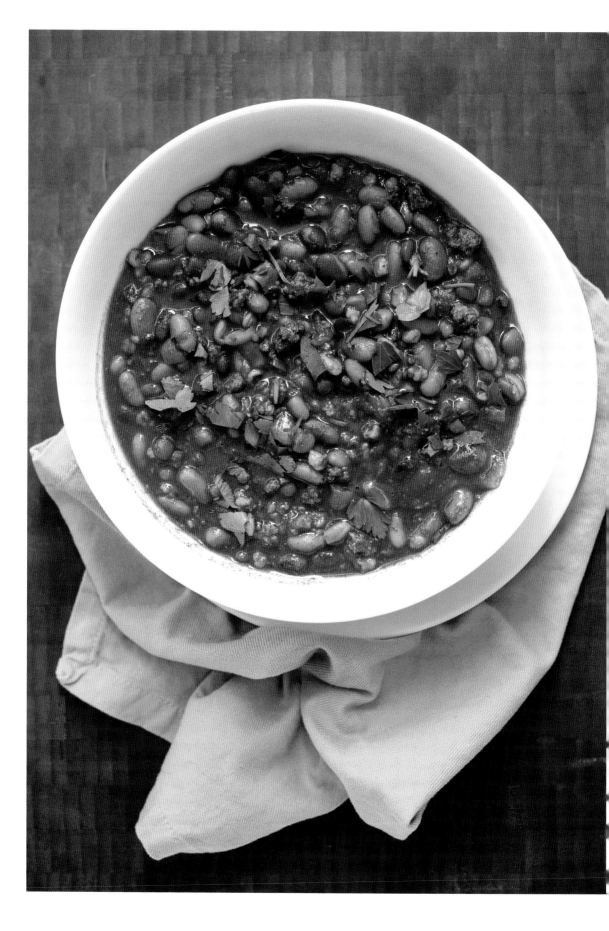

Freezer and Pantry Slow-Cooker Stew

SERVES 6

This adaptable method of using your slow cooker allows you to get a delicious meal out of things you have lying about in your freezer and pantry. As such, it is more of a road map than a recipe, but whatever combination of ingredients you choose, you will have a hearty meal without a trip to the store. I am counting on most everyone having these basics lying about. The Parmesan rind is something I keep in a bag in the freezer after I've used all the cheese. It is a great addition to any soup or stew—like a slow-release umami bomb! Some cheese counters sell them, too.

1 tablespoon canola oil
1 onion, chopped
1 pound ground meat, such as beef, turkey, or sausage (casings removed)
2 (15-ounce) cans beans, drained and rinsed
½ cup dried lentils or split peas
½ cup grains, such as barley, rice, farro, or wheat berries

1 (28-ounce) can tomatoes (whole, chopped, diced, or purée, or a jar of spaghetti sauce)
1 (32-ounce) box stock, whatever flavor you have around, or 1 quart water
Pinch red pepper flakes
1 large piece Parmesan rind (optional)
Kosher salt and freshly ground black pepper, to taste

In a medium nonstick skillet set over medium-high heat, heat the oil until it shimmers. Add the onion and sauté until it is golden brown. Transfer the onions to a slow cooker. In same pan, cook the ground meat until well browned. Drain off and discard the excess fat and juice and add the cooked meat to the slow cooker.

Add the beans, lentils, and grains and stir until well mixed. Add the tomatoes with their juices, stock, and red pepper flakes, stirring until combined. Add the Parmesan rind, if using. Turn the slow cooker to high and let cook for 4 hours.

Taste and add salt and pepper as needed. Serve hot.

> **NOTE:** You can add any leftover cooked vegetables you want to use up in the last hour of cooking—ditto for fresh herbs. If you have leftover wine, add it at the beginning of cooking.

Mediterranean Tuna Rice

SERVES 4

This dish may sound strange, but Stacey developed it in college after getting her first rice cooker. It is an unusual combination but good for you, filling, and very inexpensive to pull together. And if you have a rice cooker, it is a terrific meal when you don't have a lot of time or energy. The original version just had rice and tuna, but I have taken it out of the dorm room and transformed it into a slightly more grown-up but still very afford-able version.

½ pound peeled potatoes, cut into large chunks
    or 1 (15-ounce) can beans, drained and
    rinsed
1 teaspoon kosher salt, plus more as needed
2 tablespoons white wine vinegar
6 tablespoons extra virgin olive oil
1 teaspoon dried oregano

½ teaspoon freshly ground black pepper
4 cups cooked rice, hot or warm (see Note)
2 (5-ounce) cans tuna, drained
1 small cucumber, peeled, seeded, and chopped
    into ½-inch chunks
1 tomato, seeded and chopped

In a medium pot, place the potatoes and cold water to cover by 1 inch. Add some salt and bring to a boil over medium-high heat. Cook for 16 to 20 minutes, until the pota-toes are fork tender. Drain and set aside.

In a small bowl, mix together the vinegar, oil, oregano, salt, and pepper. Set this dressing aside.

In another large bowl, place the rice and break it apart with a fork. Flake the tuna into the bowl and mix it into the rice with the fork. Add in the potatoes, cucumber, and tomato, mixing to combine.

Add the dressing and toss until well coated. Serve warm or at room temperature.

NOTE: You can use leftover rice here, but it does need to be warm. Be sure to reheat it in the microwave before assembling the dish.

Chicken Thighs with Chorizo

SERVES 8

I love this dish as a reasonably priced way to serve a crowd without seeming skimpy. The fact that it can be done in a slow cooker also makes it great for feeding a family or for weeknight entertaining on a budget.

3 pounds bone-in, skin-on chicken thighs
Kosher salt and freshly ground pepper, to taste
1 teaspoon canola oil
4 ounces Spanish cured chorizo or pepperoni, cut into ¼-inch-thick slices
1 (15-ounce) can butter beans or chickpeas, drained and rinsed
2 small yellow onions, sliced

2 sprigs fresh thyme
¾ cup white wine
2 cups homemade or store-bought low-sodium chicken stock
1 cup diced plum tomatoes
2 teaspoons Espelette pepper or sweet paprika
¾ teaspoon red pepper flakes
Chopped fresh flat-leaf parsley, for garnish

Season the chicken thighs on both sides with salt and pepper and set them near your stovetop. Heat a Dutch oven over medium-high heat for 1 minute. Add the oil and heat until it shimmers. Add the chorizo and cook, stirring frequently, for about 3 minutes, until the fat has released and the slices are crisp. Transfer the chorizo to a slow cooker and leave the fat in the pot.

Add the chicken to the pot and cook for 4 to 5 minutes per side, until browned on each side. Transfer the chicken thighs to the slow cooker.

Reserve 2 tablespoons of the fat in the pot and discard the rest. Add the beans, onions, and thyme and sauté (still over medium-high heat) for 4 minutes, until the onions are translucent. Add the wine, stock, tomatoes, Espelette pepper, and red pepper flakes. Simmer, scraping all of the brown bits of flavor from the bottom of the pan to dissolve into the liquid, for 1 minute. Pour this mixture over the chicken and sausage in the slow cooker, stirring to be sure it is well combined.

Cover the slow cooker, and cook on high for at least 3 hours. (You can also cook it on low for up to 8 hours.) If not serving right away, set the slow cooker to low and hold it until dinnertime.

Just before serving, taste and add salt and pepper as needed. Garnish with parsley and serve hot.

> **NOTE:** If you don't have a slow cooker, you can cook this meal in a covered Dutch oven at 350°F for 1½ hours.

Classic Pot Roast

SERVES 6

This pot roast is a terrific way to get some beef in your rotation without shelling out for expensive cuts like steaks. With the carrots and potatoes, it is a one-pot meal. For a real feast, serve this with buttered egg noodles.

½ cup all-purpose flour
1 teaspoon kosher salt, pus more to taste
½ teaspoon freshly ground black pepper, plus more to taste
2 tablespoons canola oil
1 (4-pound) chuck-eye roast or other chuck roast
1 large onion, chopped
3 cloves garlic
3½ cups homemade or store-bought low-sodium beef stock

½ cup red wine
3 sprigs fresh thyme
1 pound large carrots, sliced into ½-inch chunks
1½ pounds Yukon gold potatoes, peeled and cut into 2-inch chunks
1 teaspoon mustard powder
1½ teaspoons cornstarch
2 tablespoons cold water
2 tablespoons chopped fresh flat-leaf parsley, for garnish

Preheat the oven to 300°F.

In a large, shallow baking dish, mix together the flour, salt, and pepper. Dredge the meat in the flour to get a light coating and pat firmly to remove the excess flour. In a medium Dutch oven set over medium-high heat, heat the oil until it shimmers. Sear the meat on all sides until well browned, 5 to 6 minutes per side. Transfer to a plate.

Add the onion and garlic to the pot, reduce the heat to medium, and cook for about 4 minutes, until the onions are softened and translucent. Pour in the stock and wine and bring to a boil.

Add the thyme sprigs. Return the meat to the pot, cover, and transfer to the oven. Cook, covered, for 2 to 2½ hours, until the meat is fork tender. Transfer the meat to a plate, cover with aluminum foil, and let rest for about 35 minutes.

Strain the stock and let it sit for 10 minutes so that the fat rises to the top. Spoon off and discard the fat and return the defatted stock to the pot. Bring it to a simmer over medium heat. Add the carrots and potatoes, cover, and reduce the heat to low. Continue to simmer for 30 to 35 minutes, until the vegetables are tender. Transfer the vegetables to a large serving platter and tent with foil.

Bring the liquid in the pot to a boil over medium-high heat and cook until it has reduced by about one-third. Meanwhile, in a small bowl mix together the mustard powder, cornstarch, and water until well blended. Whisk the cornstarch slurry into the simmering liquid and continue to whisk constantly until the sauce is thickened. Taste and add salt and pepper as needed.

Remove and discard the foil from the roast and the vegetables. Cut the roast into 1-inch-thick slices and place it over the vegetables on the serving platter. Pour the sauce over everything. Garnish with the parsley and serve.

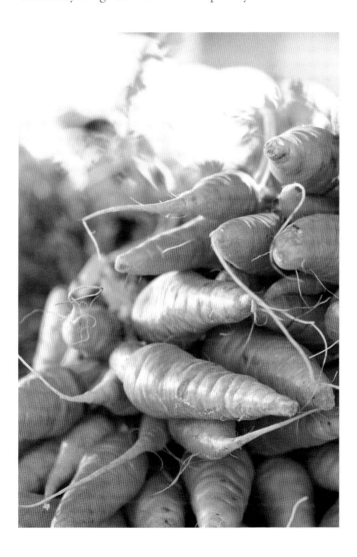

Rolled Turkey Breast

SERVES 8

This stuffed turkey breast makes for a lovely dish at a party, but it also extends the meat component, allowing you to serve many more people than if you cooked the breast meat alone. It is great served warm for dinner, but it also makes for an elegant luncheon dish if you serve it cold with a salad and crusty bread.

2 tablespoons extra virgin olive oil, divided
1 small yellow onion, minced
1 (10-ounce) package frozen chopped spinach,
    thawed and squeezed dry
½ cup crumbled goat cheese
¼ cup grated Parmesan
1 tablespoon chopped fresh basil
1 tablespoon chopped fresh flat-leaf parsley
¼ cup toasted walnuts (see Note on page 159)

1 teaspoon lemon zest
½ teaspoon kosher salt, plus more to taste
¼ teaspoon freshly ground black pepper, plus
    more to taste
2 large egg yolks
1 (1½–2-pound) boneless turkey breast half,
    butterflied and pounded to an even ½-inch
    thickness

In a small saucepan set over medium-high heat, heat 1 tablespoon of the oil until it shimmers. Add the onion and sauté until it is golden brown and tender. Remove from the heat and transfer the onion to a medium bowl; add the spinach, goat cheese, Parmesan, basil, parsley, walnuts, lemon zest, salt, pepper, and egg yolks. Using a fork, mix the ingredients well until everything is fully combined. Set aside.

Lay the turkey breast on a large cutting board or baking sheet. Season it on the top side with the salt and pepper. Spread the spinach mixture onto the turkey, leaving about a 1-inch border all the way around. Starting on one of the long edges, roll the turkey breast up so that it's tight, but not so tight that the filling squishes out the other side. If you start at the short end, the roll will be too thick and it will dry out during cooking. Using kitchen twine, tie the roll at about 2-inch intervals to help keep it together. Season the outside of the roll with salt and pepper and set aside.

Preheat the oven to 400°F.

In a large nonstick ovenproof skillet set over medium-high heat, heat the remaining tablespoon of oil until it shimmers. Place the turkey roll, seam-side down, in the skillet and sear for about 3 minutes per side, until each side is golden brown.

Transfer the skillet to the oven and roast for 20 to 25 minutes, until an instant-read thermometer inserted into the center of the roll registers 170°F. Transfer the roll to a wire rack and let rest for 15 minutes.

Remove and discard the twine, then slice the roll into 8 equal pieces. Serve right away.

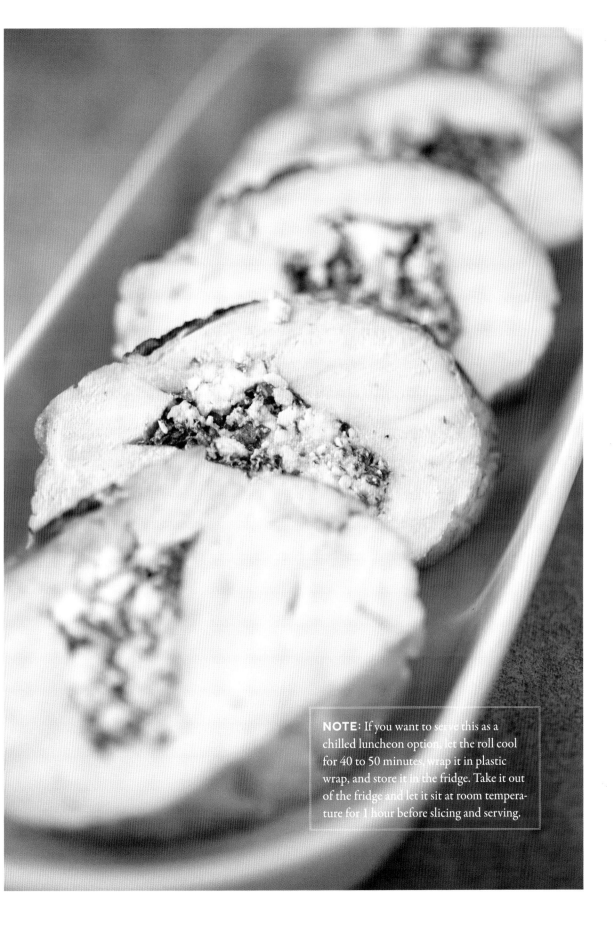

Tangerine Pulled Pork

SERVES 8 TO 12

I love this dish for both its simplicity and its frugality, but at the end of the day, it is simply a very cool take on pulled pork. Pork shoulder is a very affordable cut of meat, so it is the perfect choice when serving a crowd on a budget. I like to serve this with rice, couscous, polenta, or grits.

1 (5–6-pound) boneless pork shoulder, skin removed and most of the visible fat trimmed (your butcher can do this for you)
1 gallon apple cider, or less as needed

1 quart tangerine juice, or less as needed (see Note)
Kosher salt and freshly ground pepper, to taste

Preheat the oven to 250°F.

Put the pork shoulder in a large Dutch oven. To create a 2:1 ratio of cider to tangerine juice, use the side of the pork as a guide. Pour in the apple cider so that it comes about two-thirds of the way up the side of the pork. Add the tangerine juice until only the top inch of the pork is exposed. You might not use all of the juice or cider. Cover the pot, transfer it to the oven, and cook for 4 to 5 hours, until the meat is extremely tender and pulls apart easily with a fork.

Remove the pot from the oven and let the pork rest in the cooking liquid for 30 minutes. Remove the pork from the liquid and let it rest for another 15 minutes. Meanwhile, let the liquid settle for 10 minutes, then spoon off and discard as much of the fat as you can.

Set the pot over medium-high heat and reduce the liquid by about one-third, depending on how much there is. The sauce should have some body and not just be watery. Taste the sauce and add salt and pepper as needed.

Using 2 forks, pull the pork apart into large chunks. Place them back in the hot sauce and serve.

> **NOTE:** You can usually find tangerine juice in the fresh-juice section of a grocery store, but you can also squeeze your own. You can also substitute orange juice, but the tangerine really makes it special. On a similar note, be sure to use apple cider, not juice—juice will make the dish too sweet.

Cumin Black Beans and Brown Rice

SERVES 8

Rice and beans are a notoriously hearty and filling way to eat on a budget. The fact that the combination also creates a complete protein means it is also healthy. I love this version because it is delicious on its own or as a side dish. And since it both keeps and freezes beautifully, this is a generous recipe—half will easily serve a family of four for dinner. It also makes for a wonderful breakfast with a fried egg on top.

2 tablespoons grapeseed oil
2 medium onions, chopped
1½ teaspoons ground cumin
1 teaspoon dried oregano
Pinch red pepper flakes
2 (26-ounce) cans black beans

1 tablespoon red wine vinegar
1 dried bay leaf
1 tablespoon chopped fresh flat-leaf parsley
Kosher salt and freshly ground black pepper, to taste
2 cups brown rice, cooked

In a large saucepan set over medium-high heat, heat the oil until it shimmers. Add the onions and cook for about 5 minutes, until translucent and tender. Add the cumin, oregano, and red pepper flakes and stir to combine. Add the beans and their liquid, the vinegar, the bay leaf, and the parsley and stir to combine.

Reduce the heat to medium and bring the mixture to a simmer. Then reduce the heat to low and cook, uncovered and stirring frequently, for 35 to 40 minutes. Taste and add salt and pepper as needed. Remove and discard the bay leaf.

Serve the beans on top of the rice or mix them together. If you have leftovers, stir the rice and beans together, if necessary. Let the mixture cool to room temperature, transfer to a zip-top bag, and store in the fridge for up to 5 days or in the freezer for up to 2 months. Thaw the frozen mixture in the fridge overnight before using.

NOTE: To add more pizazz to this dish, set out garnishes such as cubed avocado, pico de gallo, shredded cheese, or chopped cilantro. Be sure to put out hot sauce for those who like it spicier!

Pasta with Last-Minute Marinara

SERVES 6 AS A SIDE

This pasta dish is a terrific and very inexpensive way to get a fast and easy pasta night on the menu, especially for a family. It works with any shape pasta, so you can use what you have lying around or buy whatever is on sale, and feel free to use generic canned tomatoes here, as you are adding enough other ingredients that you don't need to use the fancy ones. It's also a really great dish if your kids have a pal over that you want to invite to stay for dinner. If you want to bulk it up even more and get some protein going, add a couple cans of drained and rinsed white beans, some raw ground meat, or leftover cooked meats.

3 tablespoons unsalted butter
2 tablespoons extra virgin olive oil
1 large yellow onion, diced
2 cloves garlic, minced
1 tablespoon tomato paste
2 (28-ounce) cans crushed tomatoes
3 carrots, peeled
1 dried bay leaf
1 teaspoon dried oregano

1 tablespoon kosher salt, plus more to taste
Freshly ground black pepper, to taste
3 quarts water
1 pound pasta (any shape)
Extra virgin olive oil, for serving
Grated Parmesan, for serving
2 tablespoons chopped fresh basil or flat-leaf
   parsley, for serving (optional)

In a large sauté pan set over medium-high heat, melt the butter until it stops foaming. Immediately add the olive oil. Add the onion and cook for 4 to 5 minutes, until it is just soft. Add the garlic and cook for 1 minute. Stir in the tomato paste and cook until it just covers all of the onion and garlic. Add in the crushed tomatoes and stir to combine.

Toss in the carrots. Yes, they are whole; this will slightly sweeten the sauce to balance the acidity of the tomatoes without adding sugar. Stir in the bay leaf and oregano. Bring the mixture to a simmer, then reduce the heat to low and continue to simmer for about 20 minutes, just until the carrots are fork tender. Remove the bay leaf and the carrots. Taste and add salt and pepper as needed.

Discard the bay leaf but save the carrots for a cook's treat. (Give them a little drizzle of extra virgin olive oil and a sprinkle of salt and pepper.)

While the sauce is simmering, in a large stockpot set over medium-high heat, bring the water to a boil. Add the salt to the water. Add the pasta and cook for 8 to 12 minutes, until it is very al dente. Reserve 1 cup of the pasta water and then drain the pasta.

Add the cooked pasta to the simmering sauce, along with ½ cup of the reserved pasta water, stirring to combine. If there doesn't seem to be enough sauce, add more of the pasta water and continue to cook over low heat until it all comes together. Taste and add salt and pepper as needed.

Portion the pasta onto plates and garnish with a drizzle of the oil, the Parmesan, and the basil, if using. Serve hot.

Roasted Cabbage

We all know that cabbage, onions, and carrots are great for the budget, and they are certainly good for you—full of fiber and vitamins. However, people rarely think of them as delicious. I certainly never did until I tried a version of this done by Molly Stevens for her food blog. This recipe fixes that perception forever. The cabbage gets slightly sweet in the long roasting and has none of the sulfury smell or taste we often associate with this maligned vegetable. It's the perfect side dish for poultry or pork, is easy to cook, and is very inexpensive to pull together.

1 medium head green cabbage, cut into 2-inch chunks
1 large yellow onion, coarsely chopped
2 large carrots, peeled and cut into 1-inch chunks
¼ cup extra virgin olive oil

Pinch red pepper flakes
Kosher salt and freshly ground black pepper, to taste
1 lemon, cut into 8 wedges, for serving (optional)

Preheat the oven to 450°F. Grease a large baking sheet with nonstick spray and set aside.

In a large bowl, toss together the cabbage, onion, carrots, and oil until everything is well coated. Arrange the vegetables on the prepared baking sheet in a single, even layer. Season with the red pepper flakes, salt, and pepper.

Roast the vegetables, stirring occasionally, for 20 to 25 minutes, until they are browned and less colorful and some of the cabbage leaves are beginning to char. This deep browning creates terrific texture and flavor.

Remove from the oven, taste, and add salt and pepper as needed. Serve hot with the lemon wedges, if using, to squeeze over the vegetables.

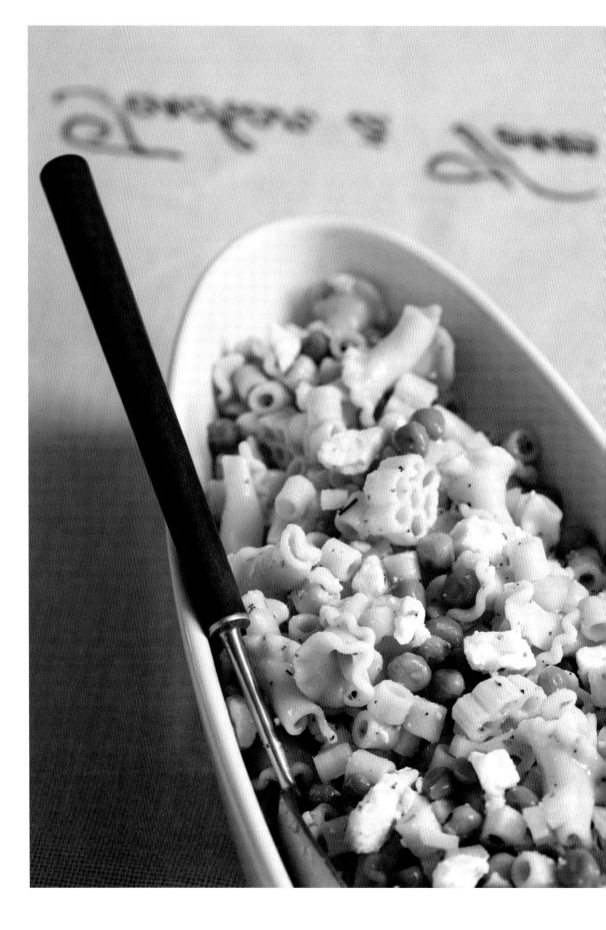

Multi-Shape Pasta Salad with Peas and Feta

You know how you always seem to have little partial packages of pasta lying around? For some reason, there's always just enough at the bottom of the box or bag to be worth saving, but never enough for a whole dish. This dish uses all those leftovers up! It doesn't matter how many different shapes you use; it looks fun and festive, and is a terrific take on a pasta salad.

Dressing
¼ cup red wine vinegar
½ cup extra virgin olive oil
2 tablespoons dried oregano
1 tablespoon kosher salt
½ teaspoon freshly ground black pepper

Salad
1 pound mixed pasta, such as penne, farfalle, and macaroni—whatever you have at home
8 ounces crumbled feta (reduced fat works fine here, but don't use fat-free)
8 ounces frozen petite or baby peas, thawed
1 cup celery, diced small
Kosher salt and freshly ground black pepper, to taste

To make the dressing, in a small bowl whisk together all of the ingredients. Set aside.

To make the salad, in a large stockpot set over medium-high heat, cook the pasta to al dente in salted water. Drain and run under cold water until the pasta has cooled but is not cold.

Transfer the pasta to a large bowl. Add the feta, peas, celery, and dressing and toss until combined. Taste and add salt and pepper as needed. Cover and transfer to the fridge if not eating right away.

Remove the salad from the fridge and let it sit at room temperature for 30 minutes. Serve at room temperature.

Dark Chocolate Pantry Cake

SERVES 8 TO 12

When I was first introduced to a version of this cake on the terrific website Food52.com, I was shocked. Could it really be that a bunch of basic, inexpensive pantry ingredients could result in a moist, crave-worthy chocolate cake? Yep. It certainly can. I've adjusted the original recipe to create a two-layer cake so that you can have an indulgent celebration cake on a budget. I also added instant espresso powder, a trick that I use to create a richer chocolate flavor in many chocolate recipes.

3 cups all-purpose flour
⅔ cup unsweetened cocoa powder
2 teaspoons instant espresso powder
2 teaspoons baking soda
2 cups granulated sugar
1 teaspoon kosher salt
½ cup + 2 tablespoons canola oil

2 cups cold water
2 tablespoons apple cider vinegar or white
   vinegar
3 teaspoons pure vanilla extract
1 cup raspberry, apricot, or cherry preserves
Powdered sugar, for dusting

Preheat the oven to 375°F. Grease 2 (8-inch) round cake pans with nonstick spray. Line the bottoms with a circle of parchment paper, then spray the parchment paper. This will help these very moist cake layers release easily from the pans. Set aside.

In a large bowl, whisk together the flour, cocoa powder, espresso powder, baking soda, sugar, and salt until well combined with no lumps. If you are worried about the texture, you can sift these together, but unless your flour or sugar is super lumpy, save the step.

In a small bowl, combine the oil, water, vinegar, and vanilla and mix. Add this mixture to the flour mixture, whisking well until the batter is smooth without lumps. It will be fairly liquid, so don't worry if it looks thin.

Evenly divide the batter between the 2 prepared pans. Tap each pan two or three times on the counter to pop any air bubbles that were created during the pour.

Transfer the pans to the center rack of the oven and bake for 25 to 35 minutes, until a wooden skewer inserted into the center of the cakes comes out clean and the cakes are pulling away from the sides of the pans. You can also press your finger gently on top to see if it bounces back.

Transfer the pans to a wire rack set over a baking sheet and let cool for 15 minutes. Remove the pans from the rack and quickly grease the rack with nonstick spray. Once cool enough to handle, run a small paring knife around the outside of the cakes. Flip the pans onto the greased rack and remove them from the cakes. Gently peel the parchment paper from the cake bottoms. Let the cakes cool completely, for about 1 hour.

Place a cake layer onto a serving platter. Gently spread the preserves over the layer. Add the second layer. Sift the powdered sugar over the top. Slice and serve.

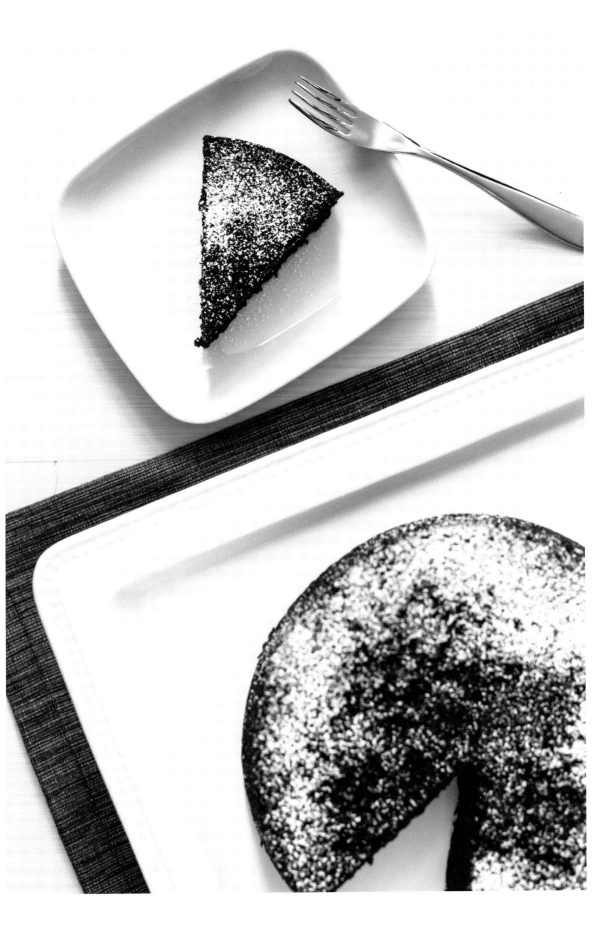

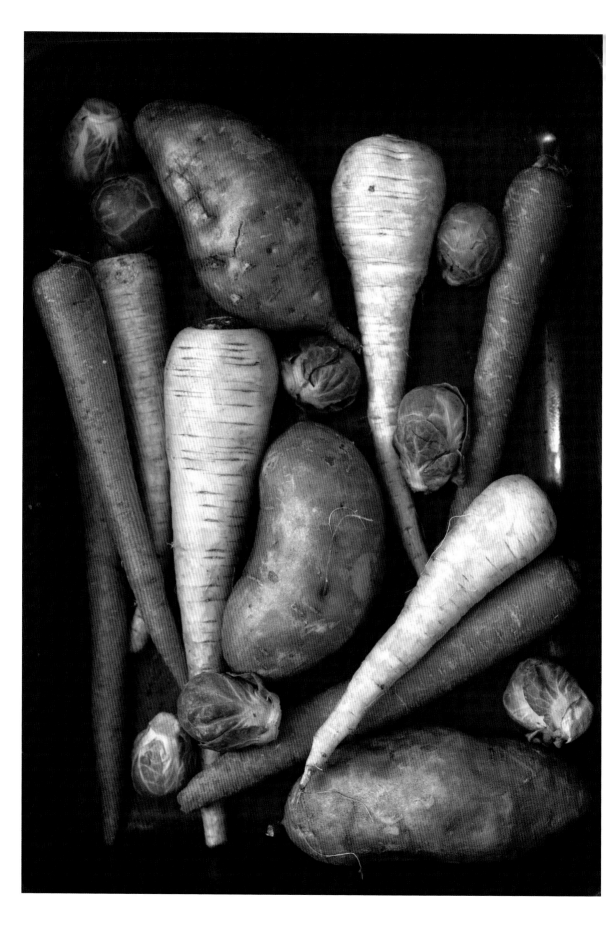

Index

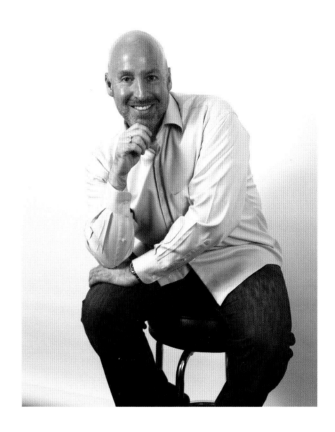

ABOUT THE AUTHOR

DR. FRANK ARDITO has been a professor of the health and wellness sciences for over twenty-five years. His contributions to the field have included numerous publications, presentations, and the development of acclaimed products and programs. Dr. Ardito was recently inducted into the National Wellness Institute's Circle of Leadership for his global contributions to the field and is the founder of The Wellness Registry, provider of the world's first consumer wellness certification: the wellness equivalent to CPR. You can learn more at mywellnessregistry.com and drfrancisardito.com.